EVOLUTION OF PREVENTIVE MEDICINE

EVOLUTION OF PREVENTIVE MEDICINE

By

SIR ARTHUR NEWSHOLME, K.C.B., M.D., F.R.C.P.

Formerly Principal Medical Officer of the Local Government Board of England, and Lecturer on Public Health Administration, School of Hygiene and Public Health, The Johns Hopkins University

BALTIMORE
THE WILLIAMS & WILKINS COMPANY
1927

In Preparation

By the Same Author

The Story of
Modern Preventive Medicine

Made in United States of America

Published June, 1927

Composed and Printed at the
WAVERLY PRESS
for
The Williams & Wilkins Company
Baltimore, Md., U. S. A.

To

Dr. William Henry Welch

the veteran chief of the Medical Profession in America; distinguished pathologist; unrivalled teacher of the institutes of medicine; profound student of the history of medicine; leader and organizer of medical education in America; and chief among those who have so widely extended the possibilities of medical research in both hemispheres:

this volume is affectionately dedicated by its author

PREFACE

During my two winters' work at the Johns Hopkins School of Hygiene and Public Health at Baltimore, my association with Dr. Welch led me to realize even more than before the importance of the historic outlook on medical problems; and I was therefore favourably disposed to the proposal that I should write an outline of the History of Preventive Medicine. There is needed in English a history of Preventive Medicine comparable in scope to Garrison's *History of Medicine;* but as this task was too formidable for me, it only remained to ascertain whether a shorter sketch might not be undertaken. In actual fact, in attempting this, I have found that perhaps nearly as much consultation of ancient volumes and old reports has been needed as for the larger task, though but little of the material thus obtained could be embodied in the following pages.

Obviously such a sketch could not include a description of public health administration, but only of the underlying principles of Preventive Medicine. From the standpoint of the medical student, of the physician, and of the general public, this limitation is advantageous; and even for the public health official it will I trust be found valuable to consider the bedrock knowledge on which administration has, stone by stone, been founded.

Beyond this, as anticipated when the book was undertaken, it has been found impracticable to deal with the tremendous developments in Preventive Medicine, and especially in Tropical Preventive Medicine, of the last seventy years. This is the less regrettable, as these advances—although constituting a fascinating story, which will be told in a second volume—are relatively well known; while the history of the earlier gropings after light, of the fights against superstition, of the even more prolonged campaign against ancient doctrine, of the ways in which error has shewn the way to progress, and of the many other events in the more remote past which have rendered the present possible, is less familiar, and it is well to have it in mind.

The table of contents shews the general scope of subjects discussed. In dealing with each period and subject I have, when possible, quoted the exact language of the writers of the past. Even with the necessary limitations mentioned above, it is evident that within the limits of this volume one cannot do justice to many of the problems discussed, and thus in the choice of material one has been obliged to omit much which might fitly have been included. But my hope is that these pages will induce others to make special study of particular periods and of the work of many of the pioneers of the past, whose names are too little known.

The present volume is complete as a study of the beginnings and earlier development of preventive medicine. The marvellous growth of scientific medicine since Pasteur has been so phenomenally great as to demand a special volume, which may follow the successful publication of the present volume.

ARTHUR NEWSHOLME

June, 1927

CONTENTS

CHAPTER I

INTRODUCTORY 1
Preventive Medicine a part of General Medicine.—Some of the subjects discussed.

CHAPTER II

THEOLOGICAL AND SACERDOTAL OBSESSIONS CONCERNING DISEASE 6
Hypotheses, theories, doctrines.—Supposed divine or demoniacal origin of disease.—Modern illustrations of this.—The King's Evil.—Fasts for Cholera.

CHAPTER III

THE ESCAPE FROM AND RELAPSE INTO SUPERNATURALISM .. 11
Aesculapius. — Hippocrates. — Aristotle. — Galen. — Witchcraft. — Astrology. — The teaching of the School of Salerno.

CHAPTER IV

THE BEGINNINGS OF EMANCIPATION 21
The value of doubt.—Paracelsus, the iconoclast.—Roger Bacon.—Francis Bacon.—The foundation in Physiology—William Harvey.

CHAPTER V

STAGES IN AND OBSTACLES TO PROGRESS 28
The foundation in Anatomy.—Vesalius.—The foundation in the natural history of disease.—Sydenham.

CHAPTER VI

THE RELATION OF SCIENCE TO MEDICINE 34

Debt of General Science to Medicine.—Physics and Medicine.—Chemistry and Medicine.—The chemistry of respiration.—Anaesthetics.—The microscope and other instruments of research.—The Röntgen rays.—An example in clinical medicine, epidemiology, and chemistry combined.—George Baker.

CHAPTER VII

THE SLOW SUBVERSION OF AUTHORITY AND INCREMENT OF SCIENCE 49

Admixture of truth and error.—Hahnemann.—Morgagni.—The rise of pathological anatomy.—Laennec.—Baillie.—Bichat.—Virchow.

CHAPTER VIII

THE GROWTH OF OUR KNOWLEDGE OF INFECTION 56

No recognition of infection by the Greeks.—Leprosy and Plague as teachers of preventive medicine.—Panic and cruelty.—Groping towards the facts, hindered by doctrine.

CHAPTER IX

EPIDEMIC CONSTITUTIONS AND EPIDEMIOLOGY 65

Season and climate and health.—Zymosis.—Instances of disappearance of seasonal influence.—Cyclical influences.—Influenza.

CHAPTER X

EARLY STRUGGLES AGAINST PLAGUE 75

Venice. — London. — Paris. — Marseilles. — Contagionists and localists.—Influence of Quarantine.

CHAPTER XI

Contagium Vivum.. 83
Fermentation.—Liebig.—Graves and Stokes.—Murchison.

CHAPTER XII

Sanitation and Social Improvement.................. 88
Roman sanitation.—Mediaeval conditions.—The struggle against filth.—Drainage and sewerage.—Water supplies.—Density of housing.—Smoke and effluvia.—Social improvement and religious enthusiasm.—Departure from earlier economics.—The driving power of Mercy.—Crime and cruelty.

CHAPTER XIII

Progress in the Eighteenth and Early Part of the Nineteenth Century........................ 101
Progress in twilight.—Plague and Typhus.—Differentiation of typhus and typhoid.—Pringle and Army hygiene.—Laymen and sanitary reform.—Social concern in preventive medicine.—Legislative reforms.

CHAPTER XIV

Poverty and Preventive Medicine.................. 113
Growth of sanitary conscience.—Panic as a motive.—Momentum for registration of deaths.—Fothergill, Percival and Farr.—Edwin Chadwick's work.—Economic motive in disease prevention.—Southwood Smith's influence.

CHAPTER XV

The Prevention of "Fever."........................ 121
Medical surveys in preventive medicine.—The Anti-Contagionist School.—Southwood Smith.—Localiz-

ing causes of disease.—Miasmata and contagia.—Historical decline of "Fever."

CHAPTER XVI

THE PREVENTION OF "FEVER" (CONTINUED) 130

History of Typhus.—Typhus and human misery.—Immobilization of infection.—Enteric fever, origin *de novo?*—Rush on Yellow Fever.—Snow's early teaching.—Simon's teaching.—Budd's investigations.—Milk as a vehicle of infection.

CHAPTER XVII

THE PREVENTION OF CHOLERA........................ 141

The unknown causes of pandemicity.—John Snow's investigations.—Budd's work.—Disinfection by anticipation.—Pettenkofer's hypothesis.—Official endorsement of this in England.

CHAPTER XVIII

DISINFECTION IN PREVENTIVE MEDICINE.............. 154

Ancient practices.—Need for differentiation of diseases.—Futile libations.—Nitrous fumigation.—Need for accurate knowledge of natural history of each disease.—Budd on disinfection in scarlet fever.—Disinfestation.

CHAPTER XIX

IMMUNIZATION AGAINST INFECTION.................... 166

A. Small Pox Inoculation.—Review of efforts against infection.—Epidemicity of small pox.—Introduction of inoculation.—Its drawbacks.—Attempt to secure universal inoculation.

B. Vaccination.—Edward Jenner.—Story of his investigations.

CHAPTER XX

The Prevention of Non-specific Infection (Sepsis)... 179
Suppuration and wounds.—Mediaeval anticipation of antisepticism.—Midwifery and sepsis.—White.—Gordon.—Holmes.—Semmelweiss.

CHAPTER XXI

Food and Drink in Relation to Health............. 190
Famine.—Scurvy.—The slowness of naval reforms.—Cook, Lind, Blane.—Compulsory dieting.—Beri-beri.—Takaki.—Food sophistications.—Alcoholism.

CHAPTER XXII

Infantile Hygiene.................................. 203
Intermingling of prevention and treatment.—The physiological side of preventive medicine.—Avoidable loss of infant life.—Seventeenth and Eighteenth century writers.—Wet nurses.—Dry nursing.—Reversion to breast-feeding.—The prevention of Rickets.

CHAPTER XXIII

Modern Preventive Medicine...................... 213
Pasteur.— Koch.—Lister.—Immunology.—Tropical Hygiene.— Tuberculosis.— Syphilis.— Light.— Vitamins,

Index of Proper Names........................... 221
Index of Subjects................................ 225

CHAPTER I

Introductory

In the history of mankind the Progress of Medicine has been the subject of assiduous study and of many volumes; and in recent years many studies have been published dealing with particular periods or with outstanding practitioners of medicine. This is not surprising, for medicine is a good index of progress in civilization. Furthermore, it is through medicine that much of the earlier progress in physical and biological sciences has been made, while rational medicine conversely is dependent on the state of development of these wider sciences.

By rational medicine is meant medicine based on knowledge of the natural history of diseases, including their causation. It is only since Harvey's discovery of the circular movement of the blood, and the chemical discoveries as to respiration, that scientific medicine became possible; but the gropings through preceding ages towards or from the light are instructive, and many pages in the following sketch will be concerned with them. To attain the most thorough knowledge of any subject, it is always important to trace its beginnings and evolution. Such a study is not only the best cure for pessimism in social outlook; it also gives most valuable suggestions as to possibilities of future progress.

Authors who have written on the growth of Preventive Medicine are relatively few; using this term in its widest sense as denoting the science of measures for the prevention of disease, and of measures which will serve to uplift the standard of health of each member of the community. So understood it includes everything which is applied in the practice of Public Health by local and central Health Authorities; and it includes also a large part of the knowledge, psychological, educational and general which is behind the work of Education Authorities, much of which ought to be in the possession of every parent and of every intelligent adolescent and adult.

In Simon's *English Sanitary Institutions reviewed in their Course of Development* (Cassell, 1890) there are admirable chapters on these underlying principles; and also a sketch of the progress of their application in administration. This latter is outside the scope of the present volume. Much information on the same subject is embodied in Colonel Fielding Garrison's classical *History of Medicine*, and in many other smaller studies, especially in biographies of the pioneers of preventive medicine; but so far as I am aware, there has been no conspective attempt to trace the growth of Preventive Medicine as distinguished from Clinical Medicine.

The object of the present volume is to show how things have come to be as they are; to trace through the ages and to separate from non-essentials the gradually increasing sum of knowledge which has increased, first slowly and in recent years rapidly, rendering possible diminished disease and enhanced health.

To give such a sketch of growing knowledge of preventive medicine, without touching and encroaching on clinical medicine at each stage is impossible; for it is largely through study of disease and its treatment that knowledge of its prevention has come; and furthermore, treatment of individual illness must always continue to be a chief means of preventing it—that is, of preventing its continuance in the individual patient, or preventing the development in him of superincumbent disease. Individual disease is, furthermore, a fruitful cause of disease and incompetence in others, either by infection, or as the result of the destitution which so often results when disease occurs in one member of a family.

It is evident that within the limits of this volume one can only select some salient features and some outstanding heroes for mention and possible discussion, in the hope that the junior physician or medical student who reads these pages may be led to study more complete histories of medicine and the lives of those who have made the present position of preventive medicine possible.

The need for selection of subjects to be discussed will be seen from the following enumeration of some of the problems of preventive medicine which have already been more or less applied in personal or public health. The growth of personal and domestic cleanliness and of personal cleanliness and chastity form an essential part of our subject. Next in order comes the growth of domestic and communal sanitation; while an account of the increasing realisation of the essential relation of housing to health if developed would occupy all the following pages.

A romantic and most important chapter in the history of health is that dealing with health in relation to food and drink, including alcohol.

Nor can the influence of air, climate and season on health, recognised by Hippocrates and Sydenham alike, be ignored.

The prevention of occupational diseases is gradually assuming its full importance; but space cannot be devoted to its growth in these pages.

Any history of preventive medicine must necessarily be concerned largely with the prevention of infection, to which the majority of the diseases of mankind are due; and there is no more interesting study than that of the growth of the idea of contagion, the differentiation of infections, and the means for immunising mankind against certain infections. The total subject of infections is too large for the present volume; and the intensely interesting growth in recent years of knowledge of the entire subject, as well as of the prevention of such mainly exotic diseases as malaria, yellow fever, ankylostomiasis, etc., must be left for discussion in another volume.

In the past preventive medicine has been chiefly concerned with the prevention of disease. It will probably remain thus in the future; and we may, in passing, deprecate the frequent assumption that there is likely to be diminishing need of active measures to this end. Furthermore, the prevention of disease, especially by the prevention of infection, must always be a chief means of prolonging life and of enhancing the standard of individual health. We need only mention the prevention of acute rheumatism, of tuberculosis, and of syphilis, as outstanding illustrations of this. But preventive medicine is becoming increasingly concerned with the physiological side of hygiene; and as the causation of rickets, of goitre, and of other diseases due to malnutrition or more subtle deficiencies in intake shews us, there is a rapidly widening field for securing a higher standard of health as well as for preventing disease. The improvement in maternal and child hygiene in this connection forms an important chapter in the history of preventive medicine.

The preceding imperfect enumeration inadequately illustrates the richness and complexity of our subject, and the severe limitations which are needed in our preliminary sketch of the history of preventive medicine. It is, moreover, clear that both the history of the prevention of tropical diseases, which is perhaps the most romantic of the problems of preventive medicine, and the fascinating story of the communal control of disease, must be almost entirely relegated for later discussion, if the study of the genesis and evolution of the possibilities of prevention are, within the limits of this volume, to be made really valuable to the reader.

CHAPTER II

Theological and Sacerdotal Obsessions Regarding Disease

The history of medicine, and especially of preventive medicine, being coterminous with the history of science, it is concerned, in its earlier stages, with various obsessions of the human mind, which successively have been elevated into the position of doctrines or dogmas.

In the process of generalization dealing with a body of facts, or more often in former days related to philosophical considerations which have taken the place of facts, certain stages are passed. A hypothesis is formed having some apparent relation to the observations. When confirmed—or apparently so—by further facts, the hypothesis becomes a Theory; and this theory becomes a Doctrine when it is regarded as embodying immutable truth.

Evidently a Doctrine which is sound is a time-saving device, obviating the need for individual decision in the special circumstances of each case; but the history of medicine is one of successive doctrines embodying false conceptions of physiology and pathology, because they have not been based on accurate and adequate observation and experimentation. In the history of medicine we repeatedly see persistent belated eddies of former doctrines, rubbing shoulders with newer doctrines, or with our present scientific knowledge.

An erroneous doctrine strangles investigation and original thought; and the history of medicine is strewn with the wreckage showing unnecessary suffering due to delay in the study of the natural history of disease and of the collateral biological sciences.

As in other branches of knowledge, orthodoxy has been the bane of progress in medical science, though each new error has usually embodied some element of truth and has perhaps formed a necessary stage in the slow evolution of knowledge.

Of the various obstacles to progress the one which stands out with special prominence is what may be called *the Sacerdotal Obsession.*

The first man was the first doctor, and probably also he was the first obstetrician. The earliest *homo sapiens* can scarcely have escaped from accident and sickness, and would naturally adopt such measures as his limited intellect suggested. Herodotus states that although among the Babylonians the chief doctors were the priests, the Babylonian sick were often brought out into the market place to elicit the views of passers-by as to their treatment.

As generations followed generations, it is not surprising that men began to associate disease and other calamities with the maleficent influence of angry gods, and that priests for long ages were the chief or the sole physicians. In the sixth century B.C. we read that during great epidemics the favour of the gods was sought by opulent banquets; also that theatrical performances were provided for the amusement of the gods. This conception of production of disease and other calamities by divine or satanic action, and the need for appeasement or diversion of superhuman wrath, runs right through ancient medicine. It was partially interrupted for a time by the Greek conception of natural causation; but it prevailed again in the early and middle ages of the Christian era. Although in the early centuries of that era monks were a chief means of preserving the medical knowledge of the earlier Greeks, monks and priests representing the only existent culture were also responsible for a relapse from a belief in the natural causation of disease which was the chief contribution of the Greek school to medical advance.

Even though risking historical orderliness, we may here illustrate this theological view of disease from modern experience. (As we deal with other aspects of preventive medicine a similar plan will occasionally be followed, in tracing a given error up to date.)

It must always be remembered that history is evolutionary; and that evidences of all different stages of mental and scientific development may be found contemporaneously. Just as in the embryonic history of mankind, each foetus passes through stages of development representing piscine or reptilian forms of life, and traces of these stages sometimes persist after birth; so in the mental and moral history of mankind, representatives of primeval, of ancient, and of mediaeval types of humanity are still found in our midst.

The great epidemic of St. Vitus' Dance in the fourteenth century was deemed to be the work of the devil. Origen (A.D. 185–254) said "it is demons which produce famine, corruption of the air and pestilence." In the opinion also of St. Augustine (A.D. 353–430) "all diseases are to be ascribed to demons," an opinion shared by Martin Luther, and hosts of others even after his time.

It was a natural development of the view that disease was directly controlled by God, that kings, as the Anointed of the Lord, were held to possess special healing powers. (See *The King's Evil* by Dr. R. Crawford, 1911.) There are traces of the supposed healing of scrofula by the King's touch as early as the reign of Edward the Confessor (A.D. 1042–1066). In the twelfth century King's Evil (Morbus regius) had become a current designation of scrofula in France. In the reign of Charles I, Sir Thomas Browne, the author of *Religio Medici*, sent children to be "touched" by the King; and in Charles II's time, distinguished scientific men like Boyle, Halley, Newton and Wren believed in the efficacy of the "touch." In 1712 Queen Anne touched Samuel Johnson, with 200 others in St. James's Palace; but "he carried with him to the grave" his defective vision as "abiding testimony of Anne's ineffectual handiwork."

One further illustration may be given showing

advance in enlightenment, along with persistent ignorant credulity in another section of the population.

In 1853, when cholera, which had previously devastated Great Britain, was once more threatened, the Presbytery of Edinburgh wrote to Lord Palmerston, then Home Secretary, suggesting that "in the circumstances a national fast should be appointed on royal authority." In his answer the Home Secretary made a statement which shews the realization of the fact that epidemics are governed by natural laws. He wrote: "The weal or woe of mankind depends upon the observance or neglect of those laws. . . . ."

He further emphasized that activity in the direction of purification of towns was preferable to humiliation, adding:

> The best course which the people of this country can pursue to deserve that the further progress of the cholera should be stayed will be to employ the interval that will elapse between the present time and the beginning of next spring, in planning and executing measures by which those portions of their towns which are inhabited by the poorer classes, and which from the nature of things must most need purification and improvement, may be freed from those causes and sources of contagion, which, if allowed to remain, will probably breed pestilence, and be fruitful in death in spite of the prayers and fastings of a united but inactive people.

CHAPTER III

The Escape from and Relapse into Supernaturalism

In the ancient world and right through the Middle Ages of the Christian era, the belief in the supernatural origin of disease persisted, and no real advance was possible in medical or general science so long as this belief dominated mankind. But in the heyday of Greek civilization there was partial release from this bondage. It was the great achievement of the Greek school that it threw off the fetters of supernaturalism in relation to disease. For long the origin of the medical art had been attributed to Esculapius, the son of Apollo and the nymph Coronis. He is reputed to have become so proficient in the healing art that Pluto accused him of diminishing the number of shades in Hades, and he was destroyed by a thunderbolt by Zeus. His successors, the Asclepiads, further developed the art; among the temples devoted to it, that of Epidauros being the most famous.

Even before the birth of Hippocrates (at Cos B.C. 460) the art of preventive medicine, so far as it is concerned with physical development, had progressed, as shown by the Grecian gymnasium with its wrestling, games, baths, etc. But scientific medicine was first voiced by Hippocrates. He made observation the foundation of medicine, recognizing disease as a part of the processes of nature, and he appears first to have grasped the great healing powers of nature (*vis medicatrix naturæ*). The assertion of the sovereignity of nature over medical science, which was the brilliant anticipation of modern medicine by Hippocrates, did not mean the adequacy of nature for the cure of disease; and Hippocrates was emphatic as to the efficacy of the medical art. But he recognized the importance of knowing the natural history of each acute disease, thus being the forerunner of the English Sydenham in the seventeenth century. Sydenham characterized Hippocrates as the "Divine old man," and our association of the two names is not fortuitous.

The doctrine of Hippocrates eliminated priests and astrologers from legitimate concern with medicine. For Galen quoted him as saying: "Our natures are the healers of our diseases;" and in his *De Aere, aquis, et locis* Hippocrates said: "No disease comes from the Gods, one more than another, each acknowledging its own natural and manifest cause." Not the least of Hippocrates' services to mankind was his high standard of medical ethics. The head of the family, Hippocrates said, must be "assured of the physician's discretion and integrity." The physician is described by him as one "who, esteeming all the wretched as equals, as all men are equals in the eyes of the Divine Being, eagerly hastens to their assistance at their call, without distinction of persons." Furthermore, the physician "speaks to his patients with mildness, listens to them with attention, bears with their impatience, and inspires them with that confidence which is sometimes sufficient to restore them to life: sensibly feeling for their sufferings, carefully and assiduously *studies the cause and progress of their complaint*" etc. (Dr. Adam's Transl. *Sydenham Soc. Transactions*).

Plato (B.C. 427–347), the great contemporary of Hippocrates, was equally emphatic as to the importance of exact observation. "To know," he said "is science, to believe one knows is ignorance." Equally striking is his aphorism: "Life is short and Art is long; the Occasion fleeting, Experience fallacious, and Judgment difficult." But Plato, unlike Hippocrates, tried to solve the problems of health and disease by intuition and speculation. Hippocrates himself and his school were not completely free from the bias of his period, for he regarded Plague as an instrument of divine wrath. He formulated the doctrine that there are four elements, earth, water, air, fire; four qualities, hot, cold, moist and dry; and four humours, blood, phlegm, yellow bile and black bile. It was believed that sickness was the result of ill-balance or disturbance of these humours, variously affected by external elements and qualities. On this foundation was built the subsequent elaboration of Galenic doctrine. There is no necessary error in the dogma as to peccant humours of the body; our modern views as to toxins, antitoxins, etc., may be regarded as their modern counterpart, with the difference that their description is based on scientific investigation, and not on intuition and speculation.

The followers of Hippocrates applied the mystical speculations of Platonic philosophy to the study of medicine, adopting the pernicious view that where observation failed reason might suffice, thus placing hypothesis on the throne instead of observation.

Aristotle (B.C. 384–322) has been aptly said to have codified Plato, with the advantage of a physician's knowledge. Throughout the following pages the importance of exact observation and of experimentation, i.e., of observation in scientifically regulated conditions, will be stressed as the only satisfactory method of advance in preventive medicine; and it is interesting to note that Aristotle was the first physician to have personal research endowed. Alexander the Great, his pupil, not only subsidised Aristotle's work, but collected and sent to him curious objects in nature and art. But Aristotle's knowledge was far from accurate. He confused the functions of arteries and veins, denied the return of the blood to the heart; and like Hippocrates confused between nerves and tendons and ligaments.

Galen (A.D. 130–201) forms the culminating point of Greek medicine. He was at the same time the founder of scientific medicine by experimentation and the leader of extreme unfounded dogmatism. No further great advance in medicine beyond the point reached by Galen was practicable, until general science as well as medical science—by exact observation and experimentation—became more advanced. Dr. R. O. Moon (*Hippocrates and his Successors*, 1923) aptly quotes an old Spanish physician in this connection: "if you only know medicine you don't know that."

Galen, through his victimisation by worthless theories, and his addition to their number, left medicine overloaded with doctrines from which we have scarcely yet escaped.

The story as to the gradual groping towards scientific light during the Christian era can only be indicated very briefly. Not in any respect in accord with Christ's teaching, Christian sacerdotalists in keeping with the then standards, perverted life into neglect of its physical conditions and even to a degraded idea of the sexual part of life. Hence in the early centuries, and even more recently, cleanliness failed to be adopted to secure goodliness, and among clerics and laics alike the "odour of sanctity" had its unpleasant physical counterpart. Perhaps much of this denial of natural and normal life was a necessary revulsion against the excesses and perversions of nature associated with later Greek and Roman "culture" (see Romans I: 27).

Although no additions were made to knowledge of the fundamental sciences, the works of Hippocrates, Aristotle and Galen in the dark 1,200 years following Galen's death were preserved by the Arabic and Saracenic schools, and in various monastic libraries. Meanwhile some of the Christian priests of the dark ages disgraced existing learning by charlatanry and imposture, their ability to add to the authority of the physician that of the terrors of the Church tempting them irresistibly to fill the clerical coffers.

Saintly charms were introduced where foul and senseless drugs failed; and saints were even specialised as being helpful in particular complaints. Abuses became so prevalent that before the middle of the twelfth century papal authority intervened to protect the public from clerical ignorance and rapacity.

WITCHCRAFT AND ASTROLOGY

The belief in witchcraft is a variant from the belief in the extra-mundane source of disease, the special powers of women with the evil eye being substituted for the caprices of a heathenishly conceived divinity. This belief was shared by Shakespeare; and the Parliament that made Oliver Cromwell Protector of England, is said to have hanged, drowned or burned 3,000 women for witchcraft; also we know that Sir Thomas Browne (1605–1682) was an expert witness for the prosecution in certain Suffolk trials for witchcraft in his time, and that the children of the Pilgrim Fathers put witches to death in New England.

Along with this must be mentioned the view that the stars in the firmament were influential in determining human fate. The story of astrology and medicine cannot be told here; but here again astrology must be looked at as a necessary element in the development of astronomy and the exact physics on which it rests. The mediaeval physician studied the horoscope of his patient; and he used the motions and conjunctions of the seven planets as helps in diagnosis and prognosis, as we now use blood counts or blood-pressure gauges or the Rontgen rays. With the Arabs Tuesday (dies Martis) and Wednesday (dies Mercurii) were the days for blood-letting, Mars being the lord of iron and blood and Mercury of the humours. Hippocrates and Galen, like Roger Bacon, considered a knowledge of the stars essential for physicians.

Thus Roger Bacon (1214–1284), probably writing about 1268, said:

> Purgations, venesections and other evacuations and constrictions, and the whole of medical practice, are based on the study of atmospheric changes due to the influence of the spheres and stars. Wherefore a physician who knows not how to take into account the positions and aspects of the planets can effect nothing in the healing arts except by chance and good fortune. This is taught by medical authorities such as Hippocrates, Galen, Rhazes . . . . and similarly experienced physicians, who know astronomy, clearly teach this by infallible proofs. (Quoted from Dr. Withington's *Medical History.*)

Although the Dark Ages were characterized by darkness which could only be dissipated by scientific knowledge of natural causation, this darkness was not entirely unrelieved. Both in ancient and mediaeval history much empirical knowledge of the science of health had accumulated. I can only mention Egyptian lore and the many wonderful rules of personal and communal health contained in the book of Leviticus; but shall illustrate the above statement by some extracts from *The School of Salerno* (English Translation by Sir John Harington, 1607, edition 1920, Hoeber, New York). This poem was probably written for William the Conqueror's son, and it had wide circulation in manuscript, and from 1480 onwards some hundreds of editions were printed. The School of Salerno near Naples emerged from the general corruption and darkness, being based on the best Greek and Arabian teaching. It must have helped to emancipate medicine from its trammels, especially as it was right in the path and was a favourite stopping place of many going and coming Crusaders. Garrison tersely describes the School of Salerno as "of purely clinical character, a *civitas Hippocratica* in the midst of monastic foundations." The general character of the work, and the then state of hygienic knowledge may be gathered from the following extracts from the English Elizabethan translation:

Ad librum

Go, tell them what thou bringst exceeds the wealth
Of all these countries for thou bringst them health.
Drink not much wine, sup light, and soon arise.

Use three Physicians still: first Doctor Quiet,
Next Doctor Merryman, and Doctor Dyet.

Rise early in the morne . . . .
Both comb your head, and rub your teeth likewise.

Long sleepe at after-noones by stirring fumes,
Breeds Slouth and Agues, Aking heads and Rheums.

Wine, women, baths, by Art or Nature warme,
Us'd or abus'd do men much good or harme.

Scorne not Garlicke, like to some that thinke
It only makes men winke, and drinke, and stinke.

Directions as to dwelling

That neare the same there be no evill sents
Of puddle-waters, or of excrements.
Let aire be cleere and light, and free from faults,
That come of secret passages and vaults.

Of washing of your hands much good doth rise,
Tis wholesome, cleanely, and relieves your eyes.
Tis good a Goat or Camel's milk to drinke,
Cowes milke and sheepes doe well, but yet an Asses
Is best of all, and all the other passes.

By Figges are lice ingendered, Lust provoken.

Foure humors reigne within our bodies wholly,
And these compared to foure Elements,
The Sanguine, Choller, Flegme, and Melancholy
Against these severall humors overflowing. . . . .
Of seventy to seventeene, if blood abound
The opening of a veine is healthfull found.

Three speciall Months (September, April, May)
There are, in which 'tis good to ope a veine;
In these 3 Months the Moone beares greatest sway.

To bleed doth cheere the pensive, and remove
The raging furies bred by burning love.

A further example shewing that mediaeval darkness was not absolute and universal is shewn in De Mandeville's partial anticipation of antiseptic surgery (page 180).

CHAPTER IV

The Beginning of Emancipation

The reign of Galen and the more evil rule of superstitition were gradually undermined. As a necessary preliminary to investigation there was the instillation of doubt. This was well expressed by Abelard (1079–1142), a bold theologian of the 12th century in the following words:

> Dubitando enim ad inquisitionem venimus,
> inquirendo veritatem percipimus

In contrast with this scientific attitude may be quoted the words forced from Galileo (1564–1642) by the Inquisition.

> Perish all physical science rather than
> one article of the Faith be lost.

Paracelsus (1491–1541), when a professor at the University of Basle publicly burnt Galen's works, but excepted those of Hippocrates, as his treatment was based on observation and experience. Paracelsus was in some respects a charlatan, and he finally announced that he had discovered the *elixir vitae;* in spite of which he died in his fiftieth year. He was somewhat of a chemist, teaching that the object of alchemy should be not to make gold, but to ameliorate disease. He is described by Dr. W. H. Welch (in

Vol. III of *Papers and Addresses*, 1920) as "the strange but true prophet of modern medicine, as he was of modern chemistry;" and Dr. Welch quotes him as saying:

> Away with these false prophets who hold that this divine science, which they dishonour and prostitute, has no other end but that of making gold and silver. True alchemy has but one aim and object, to extract the quintessence of things, and to prepare arcana, tinctures, and elixirs which may restore to man the health and soundness he has lost.

In the course of time, the dream of the alchemists has, however, recently been realised, if the alleged conversion by Miethe of the atom of mercury into one of gold is confirmed.

Paracelsus taught that the elements of the body are salt, sulphur and mercury. He threw disdain on the current polypharmacy, substituting simple preparations for strange and often disgusting compounds. He appears to have been the first to use mercury and antimony as remedies.[1]

Writing in the 15th century he preached a return to Hippocratic teaching in the following words, by which he may worthily be remembered: "Before this world comes to an end many wonderful occurrences now ascribed to the devil, will be made known, and

[1] The disciples of Paracelsus were known as Quacksalbers or Quacks. The name was derived from Queckselber or Quicksilver, i.e., Mercury, because the use of this drug was a distinguishing feature of this medical school.

then it will be seen that they are only the result of natural causes."

There were many obstacles to enlightenment, not the least being the fear of authority. Galileo's fate is well known. The epoch-making work of Copernicus establishing the heliocentric theory of the world did not see the light until 1543, although it had been completed many years earlier. The discovery of printing favoured enlightenment, and in English history the year 1470, when William Caxton first set up his printing press in England, is a great date.

Scientific workers everywhere were subject to surveillance and possible persecution. Thus in the sphere of religion, in 1564, Queen Elizabeth ordered examination of the cargoes of all vessels entering the Thames, so that any heretical books could be seized and destroyed; and in 1637 the Star Chamber enacted the penalty of imprisonment and whipping for the publisher of any book opposing the authority of the Church of England. In view of this it is not surprising that Harvey postponed the publication of his great work. The delay in publication of this work, *Exercitatio Anatomica de Motu Cordis et Sanguinis*, is explained in his own words (quoted by Osler in *The Growth of Truth*, 1907).

> To the lesser circulation, with the authority of Galen and Columbus to support it, men "will give their adhesion," but the general circulation is of so novel and unheard of character that I not only fear injury to myself from the envy of the few, but I tremble lest I have mankind at large for my enemies, so

much doth wont and custom, that hath become as another nature, and doctrine once sown and that hath struck deep root and rested from antiquity influence all men.

On its logical side the deliverance from authority was aided by great thinkers. Abelard has already been quoted. An even greater man, born out of due time, was Roger Bacon. He was born in 1214, the year before Magna Charta. More than any other mediaeval mind, whose thoughts have reached us, he saw the need for the study of nature by a new method. He said:

Experimental science has three great prerogatives over other sciences: it verifies conclusions by direct experiment; it discovers truth which they never otherwise would reach; it investigates the course of nature and opens to us a knowledge of the past and of the future.

In many passages he anticipated man's mastery over nature, and he first among the mediaevalists pointed the way to original research by experiment, as opposed to the acceptance of authority, thus laying the foundation of the inductive philosophy associated with the name of Francis Bacon. That he was not free from current errors (see page 17) merely illustrates the important principle that to obtain a view in due perspective each person must be judged in the light of the best standards of knowledge of his period. It is only thus that we can fairly think of Shakespeare as believing in witches, of Richard Baxter (1615–1691) as apparently justifying torture as a means to secure confession of witchcraft. Milton and John Wesley alike believed in witches.

The genius of Aristotle defined the laws of deductive reasoning, but such reasoning, while increasing accuracy of thought, did not conduce to advance of knowledge. Its limitation is indicated by the syllogism

> All men are subject to disease.
> Thomas is a man.
> Therefore Thomas is subject to disease.

The conclusion does not embody an extension of knowledge beyond the facts established in the two premises. The effect of Aristotle's philosophy, therefore, was to favour subjective analysis to the neglect of observation and experiment. Roger Bacon saw the way of escape from this morass, and his greater namesake Francis Bacon (1561–1626), in his "true directions concerning the interpretation of Nature" clearly exhibits the difference between the new and the old system:

> There are and can be only two ways of searching into and discovering truth. The one flies from the senses and particulars to the most general axioms, and from these principles, the truth of which it takes for settled and immovable, proceeds to judgment and to the discovery of middle axioms. The other derives axioms from the senses and particulars, rising by a gradual and unbroken ascent, so that it arrives at the most general axioms last of all.

Francis Bacon knew the writings of Hippocrates, for in Book 2 of his *Advancement of Learning*, he notes the "ancient and serious diligence" in recording special cases in preference to the "much iteration and little addition" of medical science in general which has been "more professed than laboured, and yet more laboured than advanced; the labour having been, in my judgment, rather in circle than in progression."

Harvey, the initiator of modern physiology and medicine, was equally enlightened. He is quoted by Pavy (*Harveian Oration*, 1886) as follows:

> The method of investigating truth commonly pursued at this time is to be held as erroneous and almost foolish, in which so many inquire what others have *said*, and omit to ask whether the things themselves be actually so or not; and single universal conclusions being deduced from several premises, and analogies being thence shaped out, we have frequently mere verisimilitudes handed down to us instead of positive truths.

Harvey (1578–1657) and Bacon (1561–1626) were contemporaries. We may note in passing that Harvey announced his discovery of the circulation ten years after Shakespeare's death. Bacon died two years before Harvey's great work was published, but Harvey had experimentally demonstrated the circulation of blood in 1613, and given his results in the Lumleian lectures in 1616.

We may speculate as to whether, and if so to what extent, Harvey and Bacon influenced each other.

Bacon was Harvey's patient, and Harvey is stated to have described Bacon's animadversions on the medical profession as much after the manner of a Lord Chancellor, but this may not have been said in belittlement of Bacon; for Bacon was described in his time as Chancellor of learning as well as of law. Bacon appears not to have mentioned Harvey's discovery in his writings, although it is the greatest example of application of Baconian principles in history.

Further remarks on Induction as a method of research are made on page 47; and it should be added here that Bacon's inductive method was one-sided, in so far as it deprecated hypothesis as a suggester of investigation and of the direction which this should take. On this use of hypothesis see the account of Jenner (page 176). Bacon's great service was in helping to release mankind from the obsession of untested doctrines.

CHAPTER V

STAGES IN AND OBSTACLES TO PROGRESS

Accurate knowledge of anatomy was the necessary preliminary to advance in medicine. This could be obtained only by dissections. Leonardo da Vinci (1452–1519), great painter, sculptor and scientist, made more dissections than any of his predecessors, and illustrated his dissections both of adult and embryonic life by drawings which are admirable. Reproductions of these are given by *H. Hopstick* in Volume II, *Studies in the History and Methods of Science.* Leonardo seems to have come near to an almost complete conception of the circulation of the blood.

Vesalius (1514–1564), by his publication of *De Humani Corporis Fabrica* (1543) inaugurated the era of exact anatomy and of experimental science. He was the first of the two great emancipators, as Vesalius and Harvey are described by Dr. W. H. Welch (page 22). There is little doubt that Harvey's discovery of the circulation of the blood was first suggested to him by a study of the valves of the veins, probably under the tutelage of Fabricius, a pupil of Vesalius. More than any before him Vesalius appreciated that we must have accurate knowledge of the structure of the human body to know its working. His descriptions in many respects

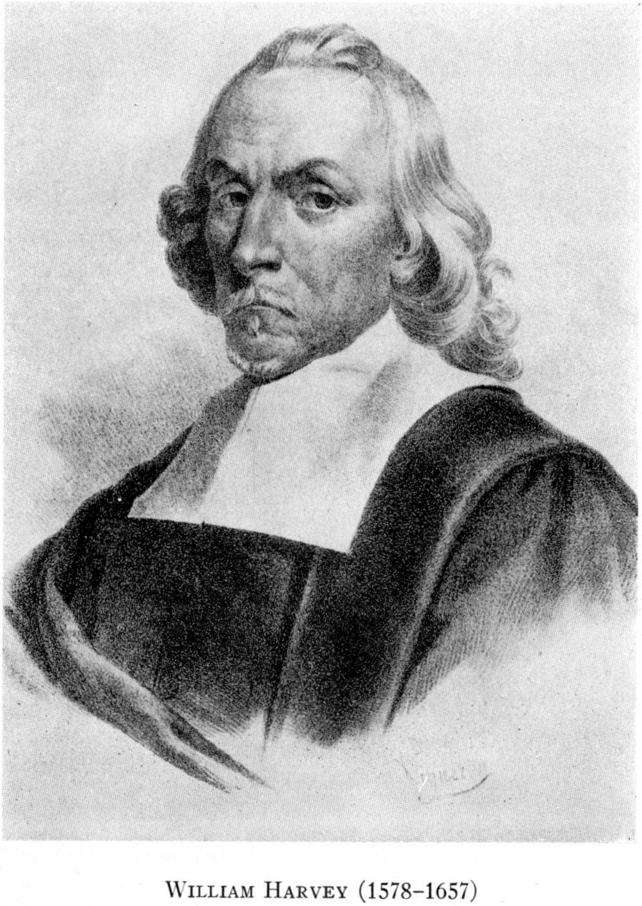

William Harvey (1578–1657)

from *Medicine: An Historical Outline*

conflicted with those of Galen; and he thus, although exposed to a storm of opposition, undermined the idolatrous adherence to immemorial authority.

The two great dates in the early history of medicine and of preventive medicine are 1543 (Vesalius) and 1613 (Harvey). These great men struck the death-knell of what Harvey described as "empty assertions, mere suppositions, and false sophisticated reasonings," which had been the cause of so much error, confusion and delay.

Although Harvey in his experiments to prove the circulation of the blood had followed out the experimental method of Hippocrates and Galen, his discovery was withstood by adherents to Galen's dogmas. Before Harvey the vascular system was regarded as a source of supply by irrigation, there being no conception of a circular movement of the blood, except partially as regards the lesser or pulmonary circulation. Even for Harvey the use of the circulation was dubious, and the rapidity of the circulation convinced him that its purpose could not be the nourishment of the tissues (Dr. R. Crawford, 1919). Two further advances of knowledge were needed to complete the fulfilment in this respect of Harvey's own injunction to the Fellows of the College of Physicians "to search and study out the secrets of Nature by experiment."

The first of these was the discovery of the capillary link between the arterial and venous circulations, and the second the discovery of oxygen and the physiology of respiration. Harvey had discovered the main fact of circulation, but working only with a simple lens he had no means of shewing how the smaller arteries and veins are connected. There followed a necessary period of incubation until the growth of collateral science demonstrated this link and fully explained the use of the circulation.

It is remarkable that Thomas Sydenham (1624–1689), a contemporary of Harvey—a Cromwellian while Harvey was the Royalist physician to Charles I —should have made the following remark, teaching us a lesson as to the uncertainty of judgment on current phenomena:

> We *may* know the larger organs of the body, but the minute structure will always be hidden from us. No microscope will ever show us the minute passages by which the chyle leaves the intestine or show by which the blood passes from the arteries to the veins.

And Harvey died without ever seeing the blood pass from arteries to veins as he knew it did. But in 1660, three years after his death and twenty years before Sydenham wrote the above statement, Malpighi, probably through a simple microscope, such as Leeuwenhoek (1632–1723) was using about the same time, saw the blood moving in the living capillaries of the transparent lung of the frog.

Even then the raison d'etre of the blood circulation was not revealed. There was needed a knowledge of the physiology of respiration, before the foundation of preventive and clinical medicine could be firmly laid. And before resuming our sketch of the progress of medicine on the clinical and pathological side, we may interpose a chapter (page 34), shewing the relation of medicine to the physical and biological sciences. But first it is opportune to indicate briefly the great work of Sydenham, which although less fundamentally important than that of his greater contemporary, Harvey, was supremely valuable in rehabilitating and extending the scope of the Hippocratic position.

Thomas Sydenham (1624–89) in England, as also Boerhaave (1668–1738) in the Low Countries, led the battle opened by Paracelsus against medical dogmas. Sydenham had fought with the Cromwellian troops, not impossibly with John Bunyan. He was intellectually a rebel, an iconoclast. He held the medical books of his time in contempt, and when asked as to the best authors for acquiring a just knowledge of medical practice, told the inquirer to read Don Quixote. He said that all disease could be described as natural history, and added:

> The only means of acquiring a correct knowledge of the fundamental principles of medicine consists in attentive observation of the whole of the phenomena of disease, and vigilant and minute inquiry into the progress and fluctuations of the several symptoms, from which alone the true and natural indications of cure can be deduced. (*Dedication of his observations on the History & Cure of Acute Diseases.*)

This inductive method he first applied to febrile diseases, emphasizing the preliminary necessity to dismiss from the mind every philosophical theory which might prejudice judgment; and having done this, the further necessity, to note down in the most accurate manner possible, the whole of the natural appearances of disease, however minute.

His writings exemplify his exact study of many diseases. He was the first great epidemiologist, laying stress on the influence of season and climate on infectious diseases. (See also page 65.) It is true that he failed to rid himself of all the hypotheses and resultant reasoning of the Galenic school. He started with the Hippocratic definition of disease as a violent effort of nature to expel the peccant matter for the renovation of the constitution. In practice, however, his common sense triumphed over speculative delusion, and modern experience has fully confirmed the value of his plan. It is only when a given disease is accurately recognised and distinguished that one can begin with any approach to accuracy an investigation of the circumstances in which it has occurred; and this is a fundamental precondition of preventive medicine.

Sydenham's method in fact was a valuable warning against premature inquiry into causation and prevention, before the characteristics of a given disease are known. Prior to Sydenham, physicians of the post-Hippocratic period followed the false clue of theory, instead of treading patiently in the footsteps of experience. As Percival has expressed it: the mistakes of physicians "have coincided with the common

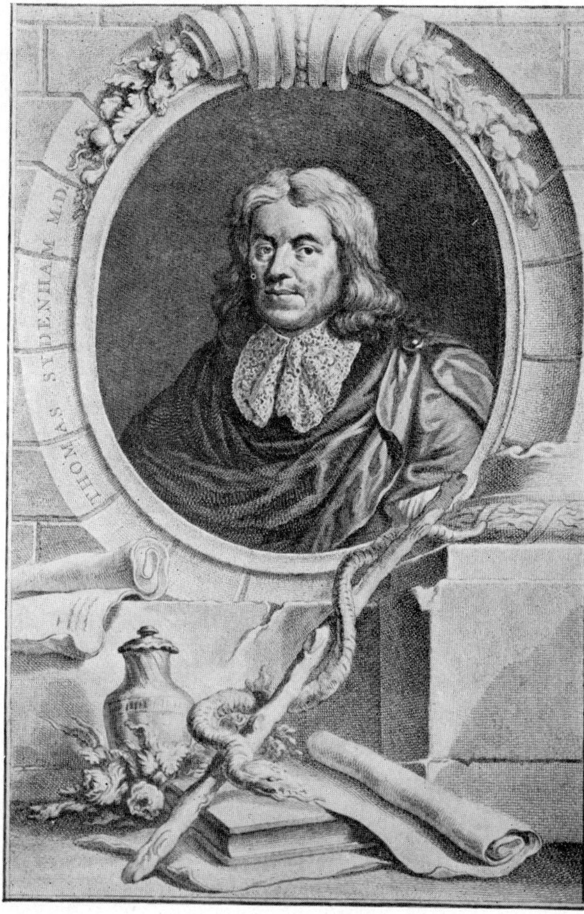

THOMAS SYDENHAM (1624–1689)

propensities of mankind, who are more inclined to search after hidden and undiscoverable causes, than to attend to the obvious phenomena of nature."

Thus while Harvey was creating the possibility of approaching the study of pathology from the anatomical and physiological side, Sydenham went far towards making the medical profession believe that progress in knowledge of disease and its causation was practicable only in the light of accurate knowledge of the phenomena of each departure from health.

J. F. Payne (in *Thomas Sydenham*, 1900) summarises Sydenham's contribution in the following weighty words:

> His great merit was to proclaim the great truth that science was, is, and always must be incomplete; and that danger lurks in the natural tendency to act upon it as if it were complete. The practical man has to be guided not only by positive knowledge, but by much that is imperfectly known. He must listen to the hints of Nature as well as to her clear utterances.

CHAPTER VI

Relation of Science to Medicine

Hippocrates had forecasted the true method of scientific investigation; and in England the two Bacons formulated more clearly the true approach to knowledge. But there was needed much greater knowledge before the fruit of Harvey's great discovery could be fully reaped; and to this end instruments of exactitude were required. In the present chapter it is proposed to pass rapidly in review some of the chief discoveries and aids to discovery in collateral sciences which have brought medicine and preventive medicine to their present position.

The relation between general and medical science is two-fold. The development of medicine has waited on that of physical, chemical and biological sciences; but in the past the practitioners of medicine have been foremost in investigation of these branches of knowledge. The latter aspect of the subject has been discussed in Sir A. Garrod's *Harveian Oration*, 1924, from which some of the following facts are taken. As an instance of the danger of disputing ancient authority may be given the fact that in 1559, Dr. John Geynes was cited before the College of Physicians because he impugned the infallibility of Galen; and he was obliged to sign a recantation of his error. The difficulties of all the great discoverers were vastly increased by the fear of authority, a fear which more or less influenced the careers of Copernicus, of Galileo, of Vesalius, of Harvey and of many more. The millstone of belief in or fear of authority weighed on would-be investigators, as well as the general standard of contemporary science; and thus we can understand how Boyle, "the morning star of physical science," spoke seriously of the thigh bone of an executed criminal as a cure for dysentery; and how Francis Bacon attributed virtues to charms and amulets, and could not bring himself to disbelieve the utility in healing wounds of applying ointments to the instruments that had made them. In this respect he resembled Sir Kenelm Digby, one of the first members of the Royal Society (1663), who invented a "powder of sympathy" (copperas), which applied to the sword helped in healing the injury caused by it. Some scientific value may be claimed for this invention, in so far as it prevented meddlesome interference with nature's efforts to heal the wound. Indeed Digby directed that the wound be left alone and kept clean. Absurd as this illustration of past ignorance may appear, it is less so than an ointment recommended by Paracelsus—a great medical reformer—(page 21), for the treatment of wounds.

Make an ointment out of moss, scraped from skulls that lie underneath the gallows, and for the other part consisting of human blood, bear fat, attar of worms and dew worms. Put into this ointment a piece of wood, moistened with some blood of the wound. By this you may, Paracelsus tells us, cure wounds of men that live 20 miles away. This remedy is also efficacious in toothache. (Quoted by Dr. H. J. Hamburger, in *Harveian Lectures of New York*, 1922–1923.)

Nicholas Copernicus (1473–1543) was a physician, as well as an astonomer, whose discoveries revolutionized physical science. Galileo Galilei (1564–1642) was a medical student when he discovered the law of the pendulum, using his pulse to time the movements of the pendulum. William Gilbert (1540–1603), who first recognised the earth's magnetic properties, and used the word electricity, was President of the College of Physicians. Galvani (1737–1798), a physician and anatomist, was led to the discovery of current electricity by investigation of the electric organs of certain fishes. Many other illustrations will be found in Garrod's *The Debt of Science to Medicine*, 1924.

A general review of the historical development of medicine illustrates the force of the saying of Hippocrates that "to know the nature of man one must know the nature of all things." The growth of natural science, and especially the investigations following on Harvey's discovery, gradually through the slow course of succeeding centuries diminished the force of Francis Bacon's dictum concerning doctors that they moved in a circle with "much iteration and small progress."

For long the science of chemistry may be said to have been non-existent, except as a part of medicine. It will be remembered that Harvey himself was not clear as to the exact object of the circulation of the blood: Sir George Ent, President of the College of Physicians, a friend of Harvey, taught that the blood serves not to nourish the body but only to keep it warm. The problem could not be solved until the chemistry of respiration was known, and the chemical fact was established that the continuance of life depends on combustion. This momentous advance was effected soon after Harvey's death. Malpighi saw the blood moving in the capillaries in 1661, and the discoveries of Boyle, Hooke, Lower, Mayow, Priestley and Lavoisier completed our knowledge of the rationale of respiration.

The substitution of the chemical for the Galenical school of medicine, which had been brought about by Paracelsus and his followers, was advanced by Van Helmont (1577–1644). He pointed out that the Galenical hypothesis of four elements, four qualities and four humours was unsupported by a shadow of evidence; he discovered carbonic acid gas and showed that an acid plays a part in gastric digestion. He possessed some glimmering of the nature of combustion.

John Mayow (1643–1675), who practised medicine at Bath, came only one step short in the complete explanation of combustion and respiration. He stated his conclusion that respiration and combustion are analogous phenomena. But for his early death the discovery of oxygen might have occurred one hundred years earlier. Lower in 1669 recognised that the change of colour of the blood in the lungs is due to the inspired air. In 1772 Priestley (1733–1804) in England discovered oxygen by heating red oxide of mercury, and shewed that a mouse could breathe this gas. Lavoisier (1743–1794) followed up this discovery, which was made independently in the same year by Scheele. He combined mercury and oxygen, and shewed that oxidation is a synthesis, and that an animal could not breathe in the nitrogen left after the oxygen had combined with mercury; thus he proved that combustion is combination with oxygen, and inferred that air owes its vital property to oxygen. He also found by burning carbon in a closed receptacle that the oxygen is consumed and is replaced by carbonic acid gas. He may therefore be awarded the honour of formulating the chemical theory of respiration, and by completing Harvey's work of inaugurating the modern era of physiology. Alchemy cannot be said to have been completely overthrown until Lavoisier thus demolished the phlogistic theory of Stahl. In 1783 Cavendish discovered the composition of water. His experiments were repeated by Lavoisier, who announced that the explosion of a mixture of inflammable and common air produces water.

To trace the subsequent dependence of medicine and preventive medicine on the physical and chemical sciences would be impossible in a few pages; but, although these and other items may be mentioned in later chapters, it is convenient to enumerate here some points in which health has depended on physical and chemical knowledge. The dependence of health on biological and especially on entomological and protozoological knowledge must be separately considered.

The progress of science in recent years has come largely through mechanical aids to vision. Of such aids the microscope has been essential to medical progress. Reference has already been made to Malphighi's discovery of the capillary circulation by observation with simple lenses. The growth of knowledge of normal and morbid histology,—that is, microscopic anatomy,—accurate knowledge of parasites, and even our knowledge of disease-causation opened out by bacteriology, has been made possible by aid of the rapidly improving microscope. The first microscope consisting of a simple lens was used by van Leeuwenhoek (1632–1723) to discover microorganisms; and Spallanzani (1729–1809) used the same means to refute the theory of spontaneous generation and thus sustained Harvey's adage *omne vivum ex ovo.*

A compound microscope was invented by the Janssen brothers in 1590, and an achromatic microscope by J. J. Lister in 1830.

Robert Boyle (1627–1691), (who was contemporaneously described as the father of chemistry and the brother of the Earl of York) introduced the air pump and thermometer into England. It was to him that Sydenham dedicates his first medical work on "Methodus Curandi Febres." The clinical thermometer, introduced late in the 18th century, has been invaluable in the study of fever.

The ophthalmoscope and laryngoscope have been important aids in the recognition of disease; and the discovery by Rontgen of X-rays in 1893 has been of the utmost importance in enabling more exact diagnosis of the position and condition of fractures, of foreign bodies, of concretions and internal tumours to be made.

The contributions of chemistry are to be seen in every branch of medicine. The chemistry of food will receive further mention (page 201), but the use of ammonia from gas works, of potash from France and Germany, and of guano and other products has been important in the development of increased food supplies. The fixation of ammonia from the air is leading to further similar developments. The production of sugar by synthesis is likely to prove a step to vast extensions of food supply.

In clothing the influence of chemistry has been conspicuous. Chlorine bleaching figures in this list. Besides making modern bacteriology possible, the discovery of the vast series of dyes arising out of Perkin's researches has added to the beauty and variety of dress; and so also has the invention of artificial fabrics and their wide adoption for dress materials.

In housing also the use of coal gas for cooking and heating, and the increasing use of electric lighting and heating are slowly reducing the smoke nuisance.

Chlorine has proved an invaluable means of safeguarding the water supplies of both large and small communities; and in antiseptic surgery and in chemiotherapeutics, especially in relation to syphilis, invaluable aids to the prevention of infection and of its consequences have been secured.

Perkin's production of the first anilin dye in 1856 was an essential link in the development of modern bacteriology. It is noteworthy that the early steps in this discovery were made when attempting the synthesis of quinine.

The value of analytical chemistry in the discovery of adulterations and sophistication of food, and in determining the purity of water need only be mentioned.

Reference should be made to the discovery of nitrous oxide by Humphrey Davy (1778–1829), as also to his investigation of fire-damp and invention of the safety lamp. Nitrous oxide was strangely neglected for some years as a means of anæsthesia for surgical work; but this discovery led the way to the utilisation of ether (1846) and of chloroform (1847) as general anaesthetics. The unexampled saving of life secured by antiseptic and aseptic surgery—one of the greatest advances in preventive medicine—was made possible and hastened by anaesthetics.

As a supplement to and illustration of the true principle and methods of investigation enunciated in Chapter IV, and illustrated in Chapter V by error as well as by progress, and as, furthermore, shewing the value of chemistry in an epidemiological investigation, I give here a summary of Sir George Baker's classical "Essay Concerning the Cause of the Endemial Colic of Devonshire," which was read in the Theatre of the College of Physicians, in London, on the 28th day of June, 1761, by George Baker, F.R.S., Physician to Her Majesty's Household (second edition, 1814).

This essay is perhaps the earliest description of an epidemiological investigation, pursued on scientific lines, and is an example for all times of sound methods of experimentation and observation. It was followed five years later by Captain Cook's contribution to the Royal Society on the historical three years' voyage of H. M. Ship *Resolution*. Baker begins his essay by deprecating the frequent toil to find remote and obscure causes, while those which are obvious and evident, *quos ante pedes sunt*, are overlooked; and he regrets that men are apt to be as partial to their own conceits as to their own offspring, and "seldom forget opinions at the bedside, which have been the result of much contemplation at home."

He then summarises the history of accounts of the Devonshire colic. Musgrave in 1603 had ascribed it to the effect of crude and sharp cider. Huxham in 1739 gave a full account of it, stating that it infests Devonshire each autumn, and that there was an exceptional incidence in 1724, when apples were specially abundant. Baker points out that Huxham's description is identical with that of the disease described in 1617 by Francis Citrois, a native of

Poitiers (colica Pictonum). Huxham described this colic as arising from the throwing into the blood of a very gross essential acid salt, or tartar contained in the juice of apples. Baker somewhat slyly quotes a sentiment from Huxham's paper, which he evidently thinks is applicable to this hypothesis: "sine experientiâ vana omnis theoria, bella sit utcunque." His doubts as to its validity are based on the following considerations:

(1) Clinical knowledge of the disease and of similar diseases. There is "not the least analogy between the juice of apples and the poison of lead: and this colic of Devonshire is precisely the same disease, which is the specific effect of all saturnine preparations."

(2) It is unlikely that two causes, so different in their character as tartar and lead should "make similar impressions on the human body."

(3) If tartar is the cause of the Devonshire colic, why is it that the inhabitants of Worcestershire, Gloucestershire and Herefordshire, who drink much cider, do not suffer from colic? And why do lead miners receive such benefit from cream of tartar, which is supposed to cause colic? Why is colic no longer epidemic in Poitou, the local wine still being drunk?

To sum up, Baker arrived at the preliminary conclusion that the cause of the Devonshire colic was "not to be sought in the pure cyder; but in some either fraudulent or accidental adulteration."

This was all in accord with the true method of

investigation. The facts had been carefully examined in a preliminary fashion. Current views had been subjected to comparison with known facts and found wanting. The investigator made a preliminary hypothesis as above. This hypothesis was backed up by his accurate clinical knowledge, and by the improbability that another cause than lead would produce the symptoms shewn alike in the Devonshire victims of the colic and in the victims of lead poisoning elsewhere.

There was now necessitated an accurate detailed investigation, followed by an analysis of all facts bearing on the disease. This inquiry Baker made.

First, he found that the colic was common throughout Devon, and "particularly infests those parts of the county where the greatest quantities of cyder are made." Furthermore, it was more common in Devon than in other parts of England. He ascertained that from September, 1762, to July 6th, 1767—285 patients had been admitted with colic and paralysis of the arms into the hospital at Exeter, most of them coming from Devonshire. Patients with this disease were frequently sent to the Bath hospital, the proportion of such patients from Devonshire to that from the counties of Hereford, Gloucester and Worcester being generally as eight to one.

Second, on investigating the apparatus for making cider, Baker ascertained that in Devonshire the large circular trough in which the apples were ground was composed of several moor-stones, "cramped together with iron, some melted lead being poured into the interstices." Larger spaces between the unequal stones were filled up with lead. In some parts of the county also there was a border of lead round the press, or it was entirely lined with that metal. Some farmers also put a leaden weight into the casks containing the cider made before the applies are ripe, in order to prevent the liquor growing sour. There was thus ample opportunity for the cider to dissolve lead from the receptacles in which the apples were ground or the casks in which it was kept.

In the three other counties, however, either the stones of the mills were joined together with putty; or where lead was used to join the cramps of iron these cramps were commonly fixed in the bed of the mill, or on the outside of the curb, and not in the groove where the apples are ground. Evidently no one plan was followed; but the lesser prevalence of colic in these three counties was associated with less frequent possibility of lead being dissolved by the local cider.

Third, Baker now proceeded to the critical test of ascertaining whether chemical analysis would shew lead in the Devonshire cider and not in cider from the three other counties. Cider a year old and the recent expressed must, both derived from a cider press lined with lead, were analysed, and lead was found. This was followed by a series of experiments with specimens of Devonshire and Herefordshire cider, lead being found in the former and not in the latter.

Fourth, although the exceptional cases of colic and lead paralysis occurring in the three other counties were not definitely associated with methods in the manufacture of cider like those of Devonshire, the general circumstances leave little doubt on this point. In a similar outbreak at the present day, it would be practicable to fill up completely this hiatus in the evidence.

Fifth, Baker agrees that lead may have been the cause of the Devonshire colic, but not necessarily received in cider. Against this is to be set the fact that no other source of ingestion of lead was discovered; and that lead was discovered in the cider.

The truth of Baker's conclusion was confirmed by the experience of freedom from colic when the possibilities of lead contamination in the manufacture of cider were removed.

Baker concludes his admirable essay with the following words:

> May not I presume to hope that the present discovery of a poison, which has for many years exerted its virulent effects on the inhabitants of Devonshire, incorporated with their daily liquor, unobserved and unsuspected, may be esteemed by those who have power, and who have opportunities, to remove the source of so much mischief, to be an object worthy of their most serious attention? . . . . I have spared no pains in this investigation; and I am insured of my reward in the consciousness of having endeavoured to preserve my countrymen and fellow-creatures from one of the most dreadful diseases incident to the human body.

Baker's investigation on the Devonshire colic is an ideal example of how disease should be investigated. It will be noted that he did not start free from an initial hypothesis as to the cause of this endemic disease. This is inevitable in most inquiries. In this instance the hypothesis was suggested by Baker's clinical knowledge of the syndrome produced by lead in poisonous doses in painters and sometimes after medicinal use of lead as a drug. His hypothesis was that it was unlikely for this syndrome to be produced by more than one agent. This working hypothesis was the child of observation and became forthwith the parent of further observation, to check its application to the Devonshire experience. Then began the careful aggregation of evidence, whether for or against his view. The negative experience in the three other counties appeared to negative his hypothesis, until he analysed their experience more fully. He next proceeded to the crucial test. He ascertained the presence of lead in the Devonshire cider, its absence from the cider of the other counties; and he failed to find any other source of lead poisoning than the cider.

To deprecate hypotheses is to attempt to stunt inquiry. It was a weak point in the Baconian philosophy that the important part of tentative hypothesis in investigation was not appreciated. The normal human mind is rightly full of the spirit of adventure; and among other adventures it is imbued with a strong desire to find a reason, an explanation, to account for all observed phenomena. Thus hypothesis is the child of observation; its only, but its constantly present risk is of becoming the master of the situation. It is when a hypothesis is accepted as an established principle that it becomes mischievous; and it is with such improper acceptance of unproved hypotheses that the obstructed course of rational medicine has been beset throughout the ages.

CHAPTER VII

The Slow Subversion of Authority and Increment of Science

In order to be fully acquainted with the historical side of the growth of Preventive Medicine, further allusion is needed to the slow removal of obstacles and building up of truth which characterised the period from the discovery of the circulation of the blood and the chemistry of respiration to the beginning of the nineteenth century. Even yet the same process continued, doctrine based on imperfect knowledge ever obtruding itself and then gradually being jostled off the scene.

For the attainment of truth not only has it been necessary to struggle out of the quicksands of dogma; but also to swim slowly and cautiously through the breakers of doubt. In the pursuit of science doubt is the beginning of wisdom.

The revival of Greek naturalism, the invention of printing, the general rebellion against authority in religion of the Protestant Reformation and against religious and regal authority of the Cromwellian period, and even the widened outlook implied in the discovery of America, all shared in rendering advance in science possible.

Truth grows by stages, new and great truths being discovered as the result of earlier work, including the mistakes of the past.

Of some of these errors of the past Percival wrote as follows (Thos. Percival, M.D., *Essays Medical and Experimental*, 3rd ed., Vol. III, 1777):

> A list of all the follies which at different periods have been established as articles of faith in medicine, would form the severest satire on the healing art. Who can withhold his laughter when he reads of expelling, attracting, and concocting faculties; of energies, sympathies, antipathies, idiosyncrasies, and occult causes; of the body being nothing but salt, sulphur and mercury; of man being a microcosm, and uniting in his frame the motion of the stars, the nature of the earth, of water, air, all vegetables and minerals, the constellations, and the four winds. Yet ridiculous as these several tenets may appear, they have given rise to sects, have been espoused with warmth, and defended with acrimony.

Hahnemann (1755–1843) may be regarded as having helped in clearing away some of the mischievous doctrines of the past. Up to his day physicians were victims of doctrines which prescribed excessive doses of alcohol in disease, or which made phlebotomy almost as great a danger to the majority of patients as their intrinsic disease. Rush, called the American Sydenham, (p. 134) is stated by Welch to have described the lancet as *magnum donum Dei*. In the reaction against these extremes Hahnemann played a part, condemning all heroic treatment, whether by bleeding, emetics, purgatives, sialogogues, diaphoretics, diuretics, setons, or blisters, for the eradication of disease. Had he stopped at this point he would have been a great benefactor; but for the current theories of plethora, morbid matter, or acidities he substituted another equally unfounded in pathology. Pathology and morbid anatomy he rejected, regarding disease as the result of the "derangement of the spiritual body that animates the human body." His theory of *similia similibus curantur* was an unbased hypothesis, and his view as to the value of minute doses of drugs was valuable in the main because it left nature undisturbed by drastic medical intervention.

It is not surprising that in view of the various theories of the centuries following Harvey, the œther of Hoffmann, the solidism of Cullen, the views of iatro-chemical and iatro-physical schools, for accounts of which reference must be made elsewhere, John Morley should have said in his volume on Voltaire: "For all the Systems we see only dismal tracts of medical darkness, we hear only the humming of the doctors, as they serve forth to men thirsting after knowledge, the draff of a medical superstitition."

Molière's satirical picture of a physician illustrates one phase of the position in his time (1622–1673).

> Above everything, that which pleases me in him, and in which he follows my example, is that he attaches himself blindly to the opinions of our forefathers, and that he has never chosen either to comprehend or to listen to the reasons and the experiments of those pretended discoveries of our age touching the circulation of the blood and other opinions of the same kidney.

In another place Molière says: "my physician comes to see me and we talk together. He gives me advice. I neglect to follow it, and I get well."

But the pathological approach to rational and especially to preventive medicine was opening out. In 1761 J. B. Morgagni published in Venice his *De Sedibus et Causis Morborum per Anatomen indagatis*, in which, as Dr. Withington says (*Medical History from the Earliest Times*, 1894), Morgagni combined all the knowledge of his predecessors in that department, while avoiding their errors. He pointed the way to localised diagnosis of disease, and strove to connect the morbid signs with the symptoms during life; insisting at the same time on the examination of every organ as well as of the one specially implicated. Prior to the advent of pathological anatomy, disease had been commonly regarded as due to crudity or imperfect action of the humours. Sydenham, for instance, despised autopsies and regarded fevers as differing from each other as the result of the different atmospheric conditions which had given rise to their epidemic spread; and the general humoral philosophy, of which this belief formed part, prevented progress in the knowledge of causation of disease.

Morgagni's work and that of his followers made possible Laennec's application of the use of the stethoscope to the diagnosis of chest diseases during life; and indeed opened the way for satisfactory progress in every department of clinical medicine. Laennec

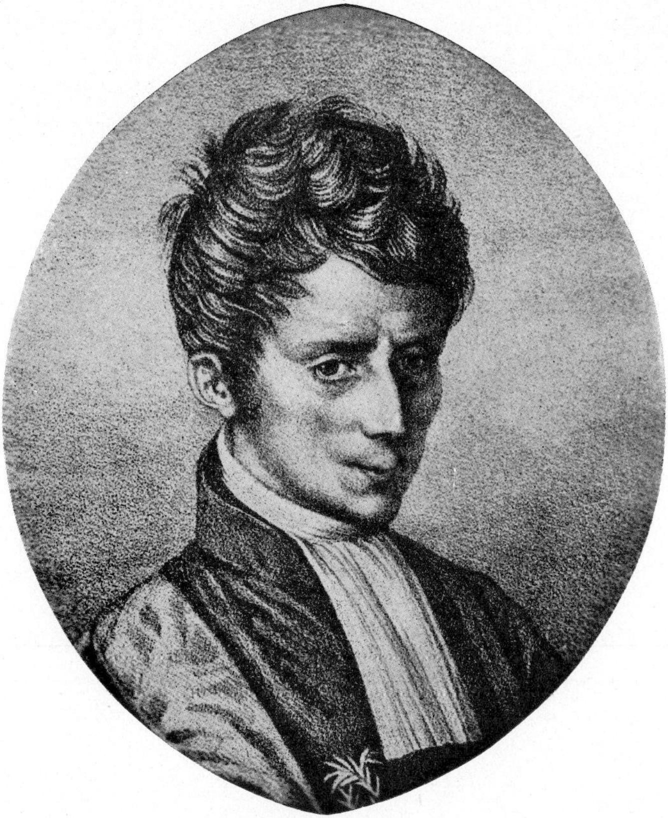

Réné Laënnec (1781–1826)

(1781–1826) was also constant in making autopsies when possible; so much so that Broussais (1772–1838),—who applied the Brownian ideas to medicine and regarded irritating agents as the sole cause of disease,—called him *l'ouvreur de cadavres.* To this Laennec retorted by naming Broussais the modern Paracelsus. But Laennec was not merely a pathologist. He related post-mortem conditions in tuberculosis of the lungs to symptoms and signs of this disease, and the publication of his work *De L'Auscultation Médiate* opened the way for earlier diagnosis and therefore easier preventive treatment of that disease. Auenbrugger in 1761 had given an account of percussion as an aid to earlier diagnosis of chest diseases. Bichat (1771–1802) was largely responsible for superseding the iatro-chemical and iatro-physical doctrines then prevalent, and replacing them by the view that disease is caused by undue interference with the functions which resist death. He founded the science of histology, shewing the special properties of the different tissues.

In England, Matthew Baillie, a relative of William and John Hunter, published in 1793 *The Morbid Anatomy of some of the most important Parts of the Human Body,* a book which entitled him to rank with Morgagni as a founder of medical pathology.

Bichat taught the medical world to look beyond organs to tissues for the seat of disease, thus advancing beyond the position established by the work of John Hunter, of Morgagni and Baillie. Rudolf

Virchow (1821–1902) taught the necessity of going further back than the tissues to seek the seat of disease in the cells of the body. Like his great predecessor, John Hunter, who began work fifty years earlier, he discarded speculation and trusted entirely to observation and experiment. As Dr. Welch has said, prior to Virchow's time, there was "no break with the prevailing ontological conception of disease as an entity, as something apart which enters the body and lives there like a parasite." Somewhat like Bichat, Virchow emphasised the idea that disease is not an independent being, but is life in changed conditions. The chief virtue of his work was in establishing the truth, *omnis cellula e cellula.* This was "the greatest advance which scientific medicine had made from its beginning."

From that time disease processes had to be judged by their effect on the cells of the affected part. Of course we now know that this view was incomplete, as there remained the questions as to how morbific agents affect cellular life. Virchow's teaching did not embody the idea of specificity as taught for instance by Laennec, Bretonneau and Villemin; who may be said to have anticipated the discovery of bacterial causes of disease. Laennec, for instance, taught correctly that early miliary tuberculosis and the caseous degeneration of phthisical lesions are stages in the same disease; for Virchow they were distinct entities.

Referring to the researches of Duclaux, Burdon

Sanderson clearly stated the later position (Life, p. 165).

> In the domain of microbiology the enzyme may in a certain sense be said to have dethroned the cell. For if, as M. Duclaux states, we can extract from the cell a substance which breathes for it, another which elaborates the simple from the complex, and finally another which reconstitutes the complex from the simple, the cell can no longer be considered as one, but rather as a complicated machine, the working of which is for the most part dependent on enzymes. . . . .

To complete our sketch of the slow subversion of authority in medicine, and its replacement by science, it would be necessary to indicate here the advances in Physiology associated with the names of Johannes Muller (1801–1859), Claude Bernard (1813–1878), of Ludwig, and of many later physiologists whose investigations have had important bearing on health and the prevention of disease. But as a part of the progress in physiology, pathology and bacteriology, as well as in biochemistry will be incidentally mentioned in later chapters, and as these subjects are more familiar to medical students and practitioners than the earlier stages of the struggle against disease, it is convenient to conclude at this point our main review of the gradual and halting progress towards the fuller but still very partial knowledge of the conditions of health, and to devote the following pages to the two main branches of preventive medicine and its application to public health, viz. our increasing knowledge of infection and its prevention, and our great advance in knowledge of the laws of health apart from infection.

CHAPTER VIII

The Growth of our Knowledge of Infection

As infection from without is the source of the main diseases of mankind, the growth of our knowledge of infection forms a supremely important part of the history of preventive medicine. This study naturally divides itself into the period before and since the discovery of the microörganisms demonstrated to be the efficient agents in producing some of the infectious diseases. It is concerned throughout with the dual struggle between the invading organisms striving to get a foothold, and the tissues of the body which attempt to resist this invasion, and to avoid becoming a laboratory culture medium for the multiplication of these organisms. The physician is the ally of the patient in this struggle, and in this capacity has important duties of prevention, as well as of alleviation and cure.

It is remarkable, as pointed out by Professor Karl Sudhoff ("The Hygienic Idea and Its Manifestations," in *Annals of Medical History*, Vol. I, page 115), that although the theory of natural causation originated with the Greeks, the Greek physicians were blind to the fact of contagion or infection. (Here the words are used as broadly synonymous.)

This is emphasized also by Colonel F. H. Garrison in his introduction to *The School of Salerno* (New

York edition, P. B. Hoeber, 1920), who points out that "the Greeks were blind to the fact of contagion, did not in the least understand that disease can be transmitted from person to person, and hence could do nothing for prophylaxis by segregation of actual or suspected cases of infection or by incineration of fomites." Their chief contribution to hygiene was in inculcating the importance of physical invigoration by daily gymnastics, by care of the skin, by swimming and massage. Nevertheless at an earlier period Hippocrates is credited by Thucydides with having driven away the Plague from Athens by causing large fires made with aromatic wood to be lighted in its streets, and by ordering strong smelling flowers to be hung up. While doubting the efficacy of such measures, they at least indicate the belief that disease may be controlled by human effort directed to the destruction of a materies morbi. To the Jews we owe two important hygienic institutions, that of a weekly day of rest, and direct efforts at prevention of infection. It is unnecessary here to indicate the relation of the relatively enlightened Jewish views on infection to Babylonian and Egyptian influences.

LEPROSY

The idea of infection developed in connection chiefly with leprosy, a disease usually associated with terrible cutaneous lesions. Probably in the Levitical regulations against leprosy, several diseases were confused, as for instance, psoriasis, true leprosy, and possibly syphilis. This is indicated by re-admission of certain patients into the community after cure, an unlikely event for true leprosy. But the Old Testament evidence of methodical inspection of supposed lepers by a priest, who can enforce temporary or permanent isolation is a remarkable anticipation of later procedures in the Middle Ages, which led to the almost complete disappearance of leprosy from Western Europe, except from Norway, where these precautionary measures were not taken. The measures stated in Leviticus, Chapter XIII, for the cleansing of infected houses illustrate the fact that by a religious route an important hygienic principle can become established sanitary practice.

In the Middle Ages, following on the vast mobilities of nations in the Crusades, leprosy became widespread in Europe. By the twelfth century isolation camps or asylums for lepers were established nearly everywhere, and there was merciless enforcement of segregation of palpable cases of leprosy. It was continued through several centuries with almost complete eventual success. This was *the first great feat of preventive medicine* in prophylaxis.

PLAGUE

The second great battle of preventive medicine was fought with but little success against Plague. It is not unlikely that the "plague of emerods" mentioned in II Samuel ii: 3, was an outbreak of bubonic plague; and mediæval history contains many details of the cruelties of misdirected isolation and quarantine of patients and entire communities, in the hope of excluding this disease. As Sudhoff has pointed out, the needs of the infectious sick, and especially of lepers, gave vast opportunities for the exercise of the "noble social blossom of young Christianity" in nursing and hospital treatment.

The two diseases just enumerated were the chief schoolmasters in making the common people realise the fact of infection: and unfortunately, side by side with philanthropy there was widespread panic and cruelty. Thus Boccaccio states that in the terrible outbreak of Plague in Florence in 1348, "when the evil had become universal, the hearts of all the inhabitants were closed to feelings of pity and humanity . . . . the brother forsook the sister, the wife her husband . . . . and even the parent his own offspring, and abandoned them, unvisited and unsoothed to their fate."

Although, as we have seen, disease for the Greeks was a disturbance of the harmony of health, and personal hygiene the keynote of Greek medicine, wars and pestilences forced upon the people the conclusion that external agents of disease existed, against which perfect personal hygiene was no protection. Lay writers like Celsus, Pliny, Virgil, assumed infection, although often misconceived, as a commonplace; but notwithstanding this for many centuries Galen's views conquered the world. His etiological system was almost entirely an elaboration of Hippocratic humoral concepts and of the theory of innate qualities. He assigned two causes for pestilences; first, a great irregularity of the seasons, and a consequent pestilential state of the air; and, secondly, a vitiated condition of the human body due to corrupt and defective food. These imputed causes, which may be described as exciting and predisposing, obviously ignore the idea of transmission of infective material.

The question of atmospheric conditions we shall discuss later.

These views with various modifications have persisted up to recent years. Thus Dr. J. Parkin, writing in 1873 (*Epidemiology: or the Remote Cause of Epidemic Diseases*, 1873, Pt. I) thinks the view that epidemic diseases are propagated solely by infection is not only erroneous, but that it has also been hostile to humanity. He instances the panic which has accompanied the devastation of pestilence, and the flight of those who might otherwise attend the sick. Until the possibilities of control emerged, such panics were almost inevitable; and history tells us also of cruelties resulting from suspicion that the pestilence was due to poisoning. In the Black Death of the 14th century the Jews were accused of poisoning the wells. At Strasburg alone 2,000 were burnt alive; and according to Hecker, 18,000 were put to a cruel death at Mayence. Parkin states that in the epidemic of cholera in Italy in 1867 the populace were convinced that this exotic disease was being spread by the air or water by poisoners. At Ardore in Calabria rioters attacked a druggist's shop and set it on fire, and many other illustrations of ignorant violence might be quoted, which bear fit company with mediaeval witch-hunting and witch-burning.

In the presence of apparently unavoidable and universal danger of mysterious origin, history has repeatedly illustrated both the kindling of the wildest passions of terror-stricken humanity, and the courage and devotion of religious leaders, of nurses, and of doctors in identical circumstances. Dr. Armstrong writing in "The Dispensary, A Poem" (1714), probably with plague or typhus in his mind, gives the following picture of the limitations of devoted help, in the centuries before these diseases had been robbed of their terrors.

> Infectious horror ran from face to face,
>   And pale despair. 'Twas all the business then
> To tend the sick and in their turns to die;
>   In heaps they fell, and oft one bed, they say,
> The sick'ning, dying and the dead contained.

As illustrating the unwillingness to accept the idea of external infection, may be given the example of Sydenham, who in none of his writings attached importance to direct infection, except in the case of plague. He regarded "acute diseases" as proceeding "from a secret and inexplicable alteration of the air, infecting men's bodies." In another place he says: "acute diseases come from God, but chronical diseases originate with ourselves." And although he writes of small pox as "infecting whole families and sparing none, of what age soever they be, if they have not had this disease already," he goes on to say "I ingenuously acknowledge, that by reason of a defect in the understanding, which is common to me and the rest of mankind, I know not the essence of this disease." On another page he reveals his real view, which is Galenical in origin: "the constitution of the air being not so inclinable to produce the Bloody-Flux gave occasion to the Small Pox."

He nowhere teaches the communicability of small pox from person to person.

Similarly Ambroise Paré taught that Plague was a wet and putrid fever, proceeding from an infected and corrupted air, and from alteration of the corporeal humours.

It is not surprising in view of the persisting ignorance, largely perpetuated by belief in ancient doctrines, that black death, sweating sickness, plague and cholera were spoken of as having each in successive ages performed their ministry by thinning out the teeming population of the earth and then disappearing from observation.

Soon after the Romans left Britain, A.D., 664 a terrible pestilence prevailed, and the following incident of the period is quoted by Dr. E. Bascome in his *History of Epidemic Pestilences*, 1851. Two kings of Erin summoned a council of clergy and laity in consequence of "a general dearth, the land not being sufficient to support the teeming population." It was decided that a general fast should be observed and that with one accord clergy and laity should "solicit God in prayer to remove by some species of pestilence the burthensome multitudes of the inferior people." An amendment was proposed that prayer should be offered instead for an increase of the produce of the land, "so that it might satisfy the needs of the people;" but this was not passed, and the record continues that speedily pestilence appeared, God's judgment falling upon the authors of the petition, most of whom perished in it.

Sydenham had described the remote causes of epidemics as "wholly inscrutable;" Cullen (1710–1796) a century later said "we know nothing of the nature of contagion that can lead us to any measure for removing or correcting it." Like Sydenham, he conceived of contagion as due to minute particles in the air, or to ferments or putrefaction of humours detained in the body beyond due time. The latter would correspond possibly to our modern conception of auto-infection; by the former was indicated so-called contagia and miasmata; but their direct convection from the sick to the healthy, apart from vicious conditions of the "humours" of the latter was not credited. Sylvius (1614–72) ascribed fever to increased velocity of the circulation. Boerhaave (1668–1738) taught that it is caused by this and by increased capillary resistance, influenced through the nervous system. John Brown (1735–88) held that fever means an asthenic state of the system from exhaustion of the natural stimuli; or from exhaustion of normal excitability. Broussais (1772–1838) held that fever always shewed local inflammation; hence the need for depletive treatment.

Our list of hypotheses and beliefs must be interrupted at this point to consider what—until recent decades—was regarded as more important than transmission of infection in the causation of epidemic diseases. Meanwhile, it must always be remembered that the hypothesis that infection is due to the entrance into the living body of special agents capable of multiplying in it and then causing disease was merely one added to the preceding dogmas as to the production of epidemics, until by careful epidemiological investigation and by the experimental production of a special infectious disease by microörganisms isolated from preceding cases of the same disease, this hypothesis had been rightly raised to the position of a doctrine based on facts. Even when for some infective diseases this position had been attained, and still more so earlier, there remained factors in the production of certain epidemics which are not fully explained by our present knowledge of the life history of the microörganisms concerned. Etiology and bacteriology are not yet strictly identical in their contents.

CHAPTER IX

EPIDEMIC CONSTITUTIONS AND EPIDEMIOLOGY

The groping out of Egyptian darkness was unduly prolonged by the doctrines as to the causation of pestilence which had been formulated by Galen and Aristotle, and which for long ages were accepted as of final authority.

Hippocrates laid great stress on variations in weather and in the character of seasons, as determining the character of epidemics: and in this particular Sydenham, more than 2,000 years later was a true disciple of the "divine old man." Much of the stress laid by Hippocrates on season and climate as causing epidemics, like his doctrine of four imaginary "humours," was medical theory, based on speculation and not solely on experience. These theories, as Payne remarks, were accepted without question by Sydenham. Hippocrates particularised a season marked by abundant showers, a south wind following drought, a hot and sultry summer with abundant rain, a humid and warm winter, extremes of cold after the conversion of the sun under the equinox, as producing severe pestilence; and Galen, followed his master as already quoted (page 14); and we exemplify a comparatively recent statement of similar views by the following extract from *Bascome on*

Epidemic Pestilences, 1851. (See also quotation on page 60).

> All epidemic diseases are to be accounted for on the principle of natural causes, viz., that atmospheric disturbance, consisting of variations of temperature, hygrometric influence, atmospheric pressure, electric tension, etc., are the exciting causes; while, on the other hand, want of light, impure air, especially from defective ventilation, in which are included malaria and all other noxious vapours, from whatever source arising; scanty diet, and habits induced by the irregular artificial life of many, are the predisposing causes, which by enervating and otherwise spoiling the system, render it more susceptible of external atmospheric impressions in the production of epidemic pestilence or disease.

Sydenham was perhaps the first to state clearly the distinction between conceptions which have often been confused.

(*a*) There was first the varying effect of a given maleficent influence (infection or other) according to the condition of the person affected by it. This conception is still seen in the prevailing idea that personal hygiene is an important safeguard against infection. If the infection received be that of small-pox or rabies there is no evidence to support this view. If it be syphilis or gonorrhoea or anthrax the same remark applies. If the infection be that of tuberculosis, on the other hand, it is arguable that personal health is an important factor; though what is often regarded as the protection afforded by personal resistance may equally well be explained on the hypothesis of varying dosage and frequency of infection by tubercle bacilli.

(*b*) There is secondly the variation of disease considered to be due to external climatic or other conditions which determine in an invaded person one or another disease, apart from any specific difference in the infecting agent. (See quotations from Sydenham, pages 61 and 76).

(*c*) Thirdly there is the phenomenon of cyclical prevalence of a disease, which constitutes the chief value of the idea of epidemic constitution. This is illustrated in Sydenham's words as follows (quoted on page 133 of Dr. J. F. Payne's *Life of Sydenham*):

> Just as an individual case of an epidemic has its proper periods, its stages of increase, crisis, and decline, so also has the constitution in general, which determines the epidemic; that is, proportionally to the time of its predominance it has definite periods; it increases from day to day in its epidemic extension; it reaches its height; it then decreases at the rate of its increases; and lastly, it dies away altogether, making room for a new constitution.

Referring to changes of type of disease, Sydenham is often quoted as describing scarlet fever as being "the mere name of a disease," so slight was it.

Dr. Payne is inclined to think that when Sydenham saw a bad case of scarlet fever he must have called it by another name; but although he may have made this mistake, there is no doubt as to the main point that scarlet fever does vary enormously in malignancy from time to time. Dr. C. V. Chapin inclines to the view that the present mildness of scarlet fever may have resulted by elimination of the more severe types by isolation of patients. It seems certain, however, that although Chapin's suggestion may express part of the truth scarlet fever does vary greatly in its characteristics. In this connection the presence in Eastern and Western countries of two varieties of small-pox, one severe and the other extremely mild, even in the unvaccinated, should be mentioned. Whether the milder form is a permanent "sport" of the more serious disease cannot at present be determined.

The ancient and persistent appeal to exceptional conditions in nature as provocative of epidemics was associated, as indicated above, with belief in their spontaneous generation. William Farr, writing in 1869, and representing accurately the then prevalent belief, said "the mere aggregation of people together in close appartments generates or diffuses the zymotic matter" (ζυμη, leaven). And again "The mere accumulation of masses of living people within narrow limits either generates or insures the diffusion of epidemic disease."

The views illustrated by Farr's statement above did not preclude personal infection as a serious factor, but they did assume the possibility of origination of an epidemic apart from a previous case of the disease in question. Some evidence of belief in personal infection is shewn throughout the ages. Rhazes (A.D. 860–932), who gave the first authentic account of small-pox, appears to have regarded this disease as well as plague, leprosy, phthisis (and epilepsy!) as communicable. He compared small pox to a fermentation. Avicenna, the Arabian, about A.D. 1037, is quoted by Hillier as referring to "many diseases which are taken from man to man like phthisis." Frascatorius (1484–1553), a famous doctor of Verona, who gave syphilis its name, in his treatise *De Contagione*, 1546, described contagion as due to *seminaria contagionum* (Garrison's *History of Medicine*, 3rd ed. p. 228), capable of reproduction; and as C. and S. Singer have shown (*Annals of Medical History*, Vol. 1 No. 1), he first clearly expounded the theory of infection as we now understand the term. To him "belongs the credit of finally and clearly distinguishing the three categories of infection, by contact, by fomites, and at a distance;" and he grasped clearly and expounded philosophically "epidemics as a result and infection as a cause". . . . his statement being free from "speculation on the barren topic of miasma."

Kircher (1602–80) after examination of almanacs and astronomical tables contended that putrid disease always prevailed when the planets Saturn and Mars were in conjunction. He inferred that these emitted morbific exhalations infecting the air and organic matter with a putrescence, innumerable animalculae being then generated. He used the microscope in his investigations; and Garrison claims for him that he was the first to state in explicit terms the doctrine of "contagium animatum" as the cause of infectious disease.

Pringle (*Observations on the Diseases of the Army*, 6th ed. 1768, page 257 (1st ed. 1752), while holding the view that a putrid ferment was the cause of the infection in Dysentery, "thinks it reasonable to suspend all hypothesis" until further inquiry has been made, in view of the dissertation published by Linnoeus (1707–78) entitled *Exanthemata viva* in favour of Kircher's view that contagion is produced by animalculae.

But in all the instances quoted and right up to the discoveries of Pasteur, there lingered the doctrine that external circumstances were chiefly responsible for epidemics and not personal transmission of disease; if not for all the cases in an epidemic, at least for the spontaneous origin of the materies morbi.

We may well ask at this point, whether there was not a substantial element of truth in the older views as to the influence of climate and season on epidemic diseases. Certain diseases like yellow fever and malaria can only prevail when temperature and moisture are favourable to stages in the life history of their vectors. In England mild winters and cool summers lower the death-rate, the former by decreasing catarrhal infections, and the latter especially by reducing the prevalence of diarrhoea. Hot and dry summers favour the occurrence not only of fatal diarrhoea in the summer, but also of enteric fever in the autumn of the same year. But recent experience shews that hygienic measures are competent to reduce or even annihilate any excess of these diseases favoured by climatic conditions. Typhus fever and small pox prevail chiefly in the winter and spring; but they are completely avoidable at all seasons. Pneumonia is much more prevalent and fatal after a cold snap accompanied by fog; and this has been ascribed to the absence of sunshine. The chief agent in causing this result, however, is the low temperature, affecting in particular those of extremes of age, with lowered vitality.

Differences of prevalence of disease associated with climatic differences are well known, as for instance in rheumatic fever, scarlet fever, diphtheria and tuberculosis; but in most instances,—and still more is this true for the tropical parasitic diseases—the difference is controllable.

Cyclical influences are manifested in a number of infectious diseases. In measles the biennial cycle appears to be mainly due to inter-epidemic accumulation of unprotected children. But in scarlet fever, diphtheria, and rheumatic fever, and in small pox, periods of slight prevalence or absence alternate with epidemic periods: and the epidemic peaks of the three first named diseases have been shewn to be highest in a series of years in which there has been an unusually small rainfall.

A most remarkable example of pandemicity at irregular intervals is that of Influenza. For some centuries this has attacked various countries at long intervals. Thus in England during the nineteenth century epidemics occurred in 1803, 1833, 1837–1838, 1847–1848 and 1889–1891. During the Great War a most fatal pandemic occurred, from which no known country escaped. Explanations of these recurring outbreaks are merely speculative; and this disease, in particular, justifies the view that even if we knew the exact bacteriology of this deadly disease, not only should we (apart from the discovery of an efficient vaccine, or other means of immunisation) be helpless to resist it; but that also we should still lack a satisfactory explanation of these recurring waves of pandemic spread. True we know that influenza spreads by personal infection; but why at irregular intervals does this infection assume increased striking power?

This disease—as also the varying virulence and carrying power of small pox, scarlet fever and diphtheria—make one ready to assume that there must occur changes in the life-habit of the causal organisms of these diseases, or changes in some force outside these organisms, the occurrence of which is unscientifically hidden in the words "epidemic constitution."

The cessation of an epidemic before everyone exposed to the disease has been protected by an attack has always been a puzzle to observers; and without discussing here epidemic curves, and the hypotheses as to their causation, the case of Plague may be cited as of interest in the history of preventive medicine. In the year 1665 nearly 70,000 died of

Plague in London. On its decline London was soon replenished by a prodigious influx of people from the country; but notwithstanding a hot and dry summer in 1666, and the fact that, owing to the great fire of that year, those parts of the metropolis which escaped the flames were crowded by "miserable and despairing multitudes," yet as Hancock states (*Researches into the Laws and Phenomena of Pestilence*, 1821), "all these causes combined were not able to restore that pestilential state of the air in London, which had already passed over the heads of its inhabitants, and which gave efficiency to every subordinate circumstance." Hancock proceeds to the pessimistic conclusion that the malignity of a pestilence abates not only "in obedience to a law over which medicine appears to have no control; but its seeds are scattered and its poison extinguished by a power more effectual and universal than all the purifications that human ingenuity can devise." In another paragraph he states as a general law of epidemicity, that when Plague begins in a new place, it begins as in the old, the same regular course, "whatever care be taken, declining with every mark of exhausted contagion." Happily the need for such a pessimistic outlook—based on the erroneous supposition that further light on the natural history of Plague was unattainable—no longer continues.

The disappearance of the Plague from London after the Great Fire has puzzled many writers. The probable explanation is given on pages 82 and 89. It was ascribed by Heberden (*Annual Medical Register* for 1808) to gradual improvement in the removal of filth and to reduction of human crowding.

Heberden's too eulogistic remarks are worth quotation:

> Our exemption from the Plague is not so much to be attributed to any accidental absence of its exciting causes, as to our change of manners, our love of cleanliness and ventilation, which have produced amongst us, I do not say an incapability, but a great unaptness any longer to receive it.

But it was not until 1762 that improvements in the City proper spread to Westminister; and yet Plague had disappeared by about 1671.

The history of plague and of cholera, as well as that of typhus and typhoid fevers, and the demonstration which preventive medicine and public health have made, that these diseases can—notwithstanding all epidemic constitutions—be reduced to insignificance or completely wiped out, should render us not entirely without hope that eventually the same may be said regarding Influenza and its congeners.

CHAPTER X

Early Struggles against Plague

Notwithstanding dogmatic teaching, people in the middle ages made up their minds that leprosy was communicable, and took precautions accordingly. So also with Plague, which unlike cholera was a familiar domestic foe, a chief enemy to life in Europe for many centuries; and the progress of the struggle towards the practice of preventive medicine can be well illustrated by giving some instances of communal efforts for the control of this pestilence. Among the earliest organised efforts against Plague were those taken by Venice, a great centre of maritime trade. The approach of the terrible pandemic of 1348 led the Venetian Republic to appoint three guardians of public health. In 1374 they denied entry to the city of infected or suspected ships, travellers and freight. In 1403 definite quarantine for 40 days was instituted, but this action was anticipated by Marseilles, where in 1383 the first quarantine station was built. It appears also that at Ragusa in Dalmatia in 1377 all travellers were rejected except after a month's quarantine. The action taken against Plague in these earlier years was an amplification of action suggested by the existent precedent of leprosy.

Sydenham regarded the infection of Plague, "when

the disease is only sporadical, as being handed from one to another:" but his general view that the character of epidemic disease may be varied by external influence is shewn by his statement that "whereas every species of plants or animals excepting a few subsist of themselves, the species of diseases depend on those humours from whence they are generated." The extent to which he recognised infection may be gathered from the following extract taken from the preface to his collected works: He ascribed disorder to the fact that

> The humours are retained longer in the body than they ought to be, either because Nature cannot concoct them and afterwards expel them, or because they have acquired a morbific disposition by this or that constitution of the air, or lastly because they are infected with some venom.

With Sydenham's views may be compared those of his contemporary Mr. William Boghurst, a London apothecary, who wrote in 1666 *An Experimental Relation of the Plague*, which was printed for the first time in the Transactions of the Epidemiological Society of London for 1893–1894 (Vol. XIII, W.S.) with a preface by Dr. J. F. Payne. In this greatest of all epidemics of plague in London 68,596 deaths occurred according to the Bills of Mortality; and Boghurst gives, in Dr. Payne's competent opinion, the best account of it. We are, however, only concerned with the very scanty evidence in his account of any measures of prophylaxis that were practised.

These are set out more fully in Dr. Nathanael Hodge's *Loimographia* published in 1672. They included the cruel measure of shutting up all the infected houses, to prevent ingress and egress, and the setting of a guard who handed in food and medicine. Evidently therefore the contagionist school of thought prevailed, as was almost inevitable in the face of such terrible mortality; though owing to lack of knowledge of the methods of infection which we now possess action was misdirected and ineffective.

A similar course of events was seen earlier in Paris in the epidemic of Plague in 1531–1533 (described in Dr. A. Chereau's brochure, 1873). The theory of contagion was fully accepted. As in London at a later period, a wooden cross was placed over each infected house; and everyone leaving this house was obliged to hold in his hand a rod or staff of white colour. It was forbidden to bring into Paris beds or linen or curtains or any other material liable to hold infection. Public vapour baths were closed for five months. Barbers and surgeons were forbidden to throw the blood produced in their operations into the Seine within Paris. Measures of cleansing and sanitation were ordered; thus the throwing of ordure from windows was prohibited. The ordinance including these and many other regulations was published in August, 1531; and some of its contents are mentioned here, and those for Marseilles in a later paragraph, as an indication of the blind method of attack which necessarily accompanied an almost complete ignorance of the natural history of plague. The terrible conditions of Paris in this epidemic have been graphically narrated by Ambroise Paré. Compulsory removal to the Hotel-Dieu of infected persons was sometimes enforced; and Paré says that many healthy persons were there lodged compulsorily with the plague-stricken.

Before referring to Mead's *Discourse on Plague*, a brief summary may be given of *A Brief Journal of what passed in the city of Marseilles, while it was afflicted with the Plague in 1720*. This contains extracts from the official registers of that city, translated into English and published in London in 1721. First, it is set out that vessels from the coasts of the Levant "being always suspected of the Plague," all ships coming thence to Marseilles are detained at the Islands of Chateaudif, and the "Intendants of Health" regulate the time and manner of their quarantaines and of purifying their cargoes by the tenour of their patents (or Bills of Health), and by the state of health of the particular places from whence they come. Fatal cases of plague having occurred on board vessels from the east the bodies were buried in lime, and the vessels placed under full quarantine. Similar treatment was given in subsequent deaths from plague in the city. As cases occurred they were conveyed to infirmaries, but many cases were concealed, and some fled from the city. The price of bread soon became exorbitant, as trade difficulties increased, and an ordinance was issued forbidding the hoarding of it. An attempt was made to oblige all strange beggars to leave the city; but as authorities in Provence forbad any Marseilliais to stir out of their own boundary this could not be enforced. Then began the proffering of panaceas. Two physicians informed the sheriffs that they could end the plague, if large quantities of wood, brushes and faggots were laid in piles at small distances in public places, and if every private person were compelled to lay a heap of them before his house; and if all these were to be set on fire at the same time in the beginning of the night—there would be an end of the Plague. This was done; "it was a magnificent sight;" but the pestilence continued. Among further provisions it was resolved that the physicians and surgeons should not demand any fee of the sick, but have salaries from the city, and be given overalls of oiled cloth and chairs, "for their more easy conveyance everywhere." All schools were closed; and later the Bishop was recommended to close the churches. All the sturdiest beggars were seized and made buriers of the dead, four "lieutenants of health" directing them. A pest-house was established. Meanwhile some physicians and almost all the master-surgeons had fled; they were ordered to return on pain of being "expelled for ever from the College of their Faculty." In the number of those who deserted the city were the two physicians, who had promised a cessation of plague after the fires they prescribed. As there was no wood for further fires, brimstone was distributed among the poor, and "the inside of all the houses was ordered to be perfumed." Much disorder prevailed because of the famine which followed, and to keep the population in awe, gibbets were ordered to be set up in all the public places.

Further detail of the multiform efforts to control this terrible pestilence cannot be given: but the above items extracted from the official account will perhaps serve to shew the efforts made ineffectually to control a disease which in Europe can now, whenever introduced, be controlled with absolute precision.

The 60,000 deaths from Plague in Marseilles and the fear of a repetition of the experience of 1660 in England, led the English Government to consult Dr. Richard Mead (1673–1754); and the following summary of his advice is taken from *A Short Discourse, concerning Pestilential Contagion, and the Methods to be used to prevent it* by Richard Mead, M.D., (8th ed. with large additions, 1722).

This was written by command of H. M. Chief Secretary of State, "in view of the sickness now in France, and fear of importation." Mead was a *contagionist*, and thus writes regarding the physicians of the older schools, who were *localists* or *constitutionalists* (if the word is permissible), attributing disease entirely to conditions of the patient or the physical locality of his life; or who believed that persons might be attacked because of fear or grief.

The truth is these physicians have engaged themselves in an hypothesis that the plague was bred in Marseilles by a long use of bad aliment, and grew so fond of their opinion, as not to be moved by the most convincing evidence. And thus it mostly happens, when we indulge conjectures instead of pursuing the true course for making discoveries in Nature.

Mead divided his proposals into (1) performing quarantines and (2) the suppressing infection here; and expressed the hope that measures taken under the first head would make measures under the second head unnecessary. If the suppression of infection already within our borders becomes necessary, he would not, he says, adopt measures formerly used in this country and more recently abroad. He regarded the imprisonment at home of all occupants of an invaded house as inhuman; and he deprecated hospital aggregation of cases once the outbreak had become large. He advised family isolation, and that those who frequent an infected house should "be obliged to carry about with them a long stick of some remarkable colour, or other visible token, by which persons may be warned from holding too free converse with them." He is clear that the utility of quarantine depends on the disease being infectious; and as regards quarantine he remarks:

> I hope I have not recommended anything prejudicial to trade; my advice being very little different from what has been long practised in all the trading ports of Italy, and in other places. Nay, were we to be more remiss in this than our neighbours, I cannot think but the fear they would have of us, must much obstruct our commerce.

Mead recommended the establishment of a Council of Health with local officials. In *The Gold Headed*

Cane (ed. 1920, p. 129), referring to the freedom of London from plague for over half a century, Mead is quoted as saying: "take my word for it, it is quarantine alone, and not any increased cleanliness on the part of the inhabitants that has kept out the plague." He was more nearly right, when he argued that it was not the Great Fire of 1666 which rid London of the Plague, for the Borough, Wapping and Smithfield, and some of the poorer quarters of London were spared by the fire. Also in Bristol where no fire occurred, and which had a foreign trade second only to that of London, the plague disappeared.

The preceding illustrations serve to emphasise the importance of exact scientific knowledge of the causation of a disease. Most of the measures cited above were in large measure futile; and could not be otherwise until there was secured improved conditions of housing, which would keep rats out of houses, and prior to the happy replacement of the black by the brown and non-domestic rat in England and many other temperate countries.

CHAPTER XI

Contagium Vivum

We have seen that, even in mediaeval times, the view that pestilences were spread by personal infection prevailed in practice, notwithstanding the teaching of venerable and orthodox authority. According to the pundits the source of such pestilences was to be found in certain special atmospheric and telluric conditions, and in disorder of the corporeal humours, perhaps aided in some instances to some extent by infection from person to person. Sydenham, for instance, admitted infection in Plague, but denied it for Small-pox.

Although Mead and some physicians as well as those in control of public action accepted the doctrine of contagion, in part at least, it was denied by anti-contagionists so recently as the seventh decade of the nineteenth century, when Pasteur's discoveries made this position almost untenable. And Mead himself, like his contemporaries, held the view that "a corrupted state of air attends all Plagues."

John Locke, a personal friend of Sydenham, in his *Ars Medica*, 1669, attacking the firmly entrenched humoral doctrines, said that he who thinks he will become an able physician by studying the doctrines of the humours, or that he will be helped in his treatment of a fever by his knowledge of sulphur and mercury

> may as rationally believe that his cook owes his skill in roasting and boiling to his study of the elements, and that his speculations about fire and water have taught him that the same seething liquor that boils the egg hard makes the hen tender.

Already the need for accurate observation as the basis of medicine was being stressed; and it is appropriate here to quote Rousseau's familiar words from *Émile* which Louis (1787–1872), the founder of medical as distinguished from vital statistics, prefixed in 1829 to his work on typhoid fever:

> Je sais, que la vérité est dans les choses et non dans mon esprit qui les juge, et que moins je mets du mien dans les jugements que j'eu porté plus je suis sûr d'approcher de la vérité.

Thus the necessity of accurate observation and the avoidance of preconception and still more of dogmas was becoming increasingly recognised.

The stages in the progress towards an appreciation of *contagium vivum* have great historic interest. Some of the stages of belief have already been indicated (page 56 *et seq.*). For long, the opinion was held that epidemics were caused by some form of fermentation; and even when it was agreed that this "fermentation" was caused by living organisms, it was still commonly maintained that these might originate *de novo*.

Robert Boyle, the protagonist of the experimental method observed with the precision of genius:

> He that thoroughly understands the nature of ferments and of fermentation shall probably be much better able than he who ignores them, to give a fair account of certain diseases (as well fevers as others) which will perhaps be never properly understood without an insight into the doctrine of fermentation.

Boyle died in 1691, only 47 years after Van Helmont, who was confident that he had experimentally transformed wheat in a bottle into mice. The ancients believed that alligators were bred of the mud of the Nile, and that, as Virgil sang, bees may be engendered in the entrails of a putrid ox. Aristotle asserted: "all dry bodies which become damp and all damp bodies which are dried, engender animal life." This belief in spontaneous generation was revived at intervals. In its cruder form, as for instance in the belief that worms may be produced by Thames mud, or that mites are created from a cheese, as well as in the more subtle form that epidemic diseases arise apart from infection, it has been current during the lifetime of many now living. The first step in its scientific refutation was taken when Francesco Redi (1626–1698) Florentine poet and court physician, proved that maggots are not bred in meat on which flies are prevented by wire screens from laying their eggs.

Fermentation, as is now well known, may be caused by non-living matter, as for instance in the action of pepsin on albumin, or by the action of living organisms, as illustrated by the yeast plant, which breaks up sugar into alcohol and carbonic acid gas; and in the earlier part of the nineteenth century the view that epidemic diseases were caused by non-living ferments still prevailed. The teaching of Von Liebig (1803–1873), the founder of agricultural chemistry, was that fermentation and putrefaction were the result of catalysis, and he disbelieved or ignored bacteria or living ferments. Even the yeast plant he regarded as non-living. The influence of his teaching persisted, notwithstanding the experiments of Cogniard Latour (1777–1869) and of Theodor Schwann (1810–1892). It was finally destroyed by Pasteur's work on fermentation.

William Stokes (1804–1878), still holding in part Sydenham's views, combatted the idea that insanitation without contagion can originate fever, but added: "the same exciting cause—at least as far as we can see it—is capable of producing different kinds of fever in different persons."

In his classical lectures on the principles and practice of physic Sir Thos. Watson (1792–1882) similar views were taught. He held, for instance, that the difference between typhus and typhoid fevers recently elucidated by Sir William Jenner in England and at an earlier date by Gerhard in America, was dependent on epidemic constitutions rather than on essential differences between the two diseases.

Even Chas. Murchison (1830–1879) one of London's

greatest clinical teachers writing in 1873 (*A Treatise on the Continued Fevers of Great Britain*) was justified in the statement that there were "good grounds for believing that contagious fevers have occasionally an independent origin;" and in deprecating furthermore the view that "if a disease can once be proved to be contagious, it cannot possibly arise in any other way than by contagion." Murchison, under whom the present writer worked as "clinical clerk," was a man of consummate skill and judgment, and the following summation by him of evidence available up to 1873 may be accepted as an accurate judgment on then extant knowledge.

> The parasitic theory rests solely on analogy and is unsupported by facts. If all contagious diseases can arise in no other way than by contagion, their germs must be both omnipresent and indestructible by time. There are certain contagious diseases, such as erysipelas, pyœmia and puerperal fevers, whose origin *de novo* may be said to be a matter of almost daily observation, and which, in fact, we have almost the power of generating at will. For these reasons and others there are good grounds for believing that contagious fevers have occasionally an independent origin.

Before further tracing the course of events up to the period initiated by Pasteur's immortal work, we may pause to describe in brief outline the groping after truth, and the successes and failures in preventive medicine which characterised the first six or seven decades of the nineteenth century.

CHAPTER XII

Sanitation and Social Improvement

Throughout the ages it has been recognised that the aggregation of people in cities is accompanied by intensification of epidemic disease and by lowering of the standard of health; and social history consists largely in a statement of efforts to counteract these maleficent tendencies by regulation and improvement of housing, of sewerage, of water supplies, of ventilation, and of food. In this chapter we cannot attempt more than to give a few illustrations of evils and of action attempted against these; but, although this chapter is thus limited, it will be understood that no study of the growth of preventive medicine is complete which does not comprise some reference to domestic and municipal sanitation and a survey of the increasingly high standards of conduct as regards destitution, cruelty and vice. These problems are discussed in many works, and the wise physician, whether in preventive or curative medicine, is conversant with these wider aspects of his daily work.

One of the chief difficulties throughout the ages has been in the removal of liquid and solid excreta, and other decomposable matter from houses and their vicinity; and a chief reason why in past centuries plague decimated populations was the abundant feeding of rats and their rapid multiplication which was favoured by the retention of decomposing food and other organic refuse in and about houses. As we now know Plague is primarily an epidemic disease of rats; the fleas infecting the rat proceed to infest and infect man, if he is within reach, when the rat dies from plague.

In ancient and even in mediaeval cities the conditions as regards filth were almost indescribable. The Romans formed a partial exception. To their chief cities they brought supplies of water through aqueducts which can still be seen; they constructed sewers.[1] They also had a system of periodical removal of refuse. Earthenware pipes are probably as old as pottery; they have been found beneath mounds of Assyrian ruins. They were used by the Romans for the canalisation of water supplies. According to Livy the cloaca maxima of Rome was as old as the reign of Tarquinius Superbus. Many of the old sewers had been water-courses. In London sewers seem to have been first constructed (*Lectures, etc., on Sanitary Questions,* Robert Rawlinson, C.B., 1876), in 1428, in Henry VI's time.

As early as 1290 the monks of Whitefriars in London were complaining of the putrid emanations from the Fleet Ditch, which had "caused the death of many brethren;" and the well-known lines of Swift (1667–1745), describing the effects of a city

[1] For further particulars see *Outlines of Greek and Roman Medicine*. by Dr. J. S. Elliott, 1914.

shower, may have alluded to conditions in Dublin or in London.

> Now from all parts the swelling kennels flow,
>   And bear their trophies with them as they go;
> Filth of all hues and odours seems to tell
>   What street they sailed from, by their sight or smell;
> Sweepings from butchers' stalls, dung, guts and blood,
>   Drowned puppies, stinking sprats, all drenched in mud,
> Dead cats and turnip-tops come tumbling down the flood.

Mapother (*Lectures on Public Health*, 1867), gives the following reference to correspondence in the first century of the Christian era. Modern difficulties make the problem here illustrated appear quite familiar.

Pliny, writing to Trajan says that through the city of Aurastris there courses a river, which is in fact a very nasty sewer, filthy and disgusting to the sight, and pestilential by its most horrible odour. Trajan, in response to Pliny, agrees that it is reasonable to have this water covered, and adds in true official fashion: "I am quite certain that, with your usual diligence, you will take care that money be not wanting to the work."

It is noteworthy that most of the main sewers of London have been constructed since 1824; and Rawlinson, writing in 1862, said that in the previous twenty years some 100,000 cesspools had been abolished. Prior to this, discharge of domestic drains and of overflows from cesspools into sewers was forbidden by law within the city of London.

Rawlinson claimed that the death-rate in London fell in proportion to the reduction of cesspools; but this, although approximately the fact, did not mean more than a partial true correlation between the two phenomena. Other factors were simultaneously at work. Both in London and Paris in large houses the latrines were generally placed under staircases. These were emptied at intervals by scavengers. It was forbidden to throw ordure into the street or river; and in Paris in 1529 during the prevalence of Plague, a special ordinance forbad the throwing of filth out of windows. As recently as 1844 Rawlinson noted that under the basement of Windsor Castle there were 53 cesspools full and overflowing; and that no window in the Royal apartments could be opened at the top.

Water-closets, which had been known before, were revived and began to be used at the beginning of the nineteenth century: and their use rendered the introduction of adequate main sewerage an urgent problem.

Central water supplies on anything like the scale of ancient Rome were slow of introduction. Shallow wells formed the chief supply for London; and the growth of London was thereby restricted to the gravel beds near the Thames where water could be obtained from such wells. It was not until 1613 that the New River, 48 miles long, for the supply of part of London with water was completed.

The housing in London may be taken as illustrative of past conditions compared with which our modern deficiencies, though serious enough, are relatively small. Up to the early part of Queen Elizabeth's reign cottages in England generally consisted of one room without chimneys. Most of the houses, even in towns, were built of wood, and chimneys were exceptional. Brick buildings only came into use in Charles I's reign, the custom being imported from Italy. As regards their interior, rushes were commonly used to cover the floors, an annual Rush-bearing Sunday being kept in some parts of England.

In earlier centuries many edicts were issued forbidding the building of more houses in the suburbs of London, which still further increased the density of population on area. We are apt to think of the crowding of several families into one house as a modern innovation; but that this is not so is shewn by the following extracts from an edict of Queen Elizabeth at the time of her "progress" in 1572. The authorities were enjoined to "forbear from letting, or suffering any more families than one only to be placed or to inhabit from henceforth in any house that heretofore has been inhabited." They were further enjoined to prevent "the heaping up of multitudes of families in the same house, or the converting of any one house into multitudes of tenements for dwelling or victualling purposes."

Following the Great Fire of London in 1666 some improvement in housing occurred, but conditions both in London and in other great cities remained terribly bad. Thus Dr. J. Burn Russell, writing about sixty years ago, of "ticketed houses"—sublet in single rooms to the poorest classes—in Glasgow, gives a graphic description of the evils of overcrowding, and of the exorbitant rents which were charged for inadequate accommodation. In these tenements, he remarks, "poverty instead of receiving discount has to pay interest," and the tenant "not only pays interest on his poverty, but on his character. . . . . He is afraid to complain, paying dearly for a bad article."

The smoke nuisance in towns was legislated against in Edward I's time, the use of soft coal in the city being prohibited by proclamation, on penalty of a fine, or for a second offence by demolishing the furnaces, etc. "wherein they burnt the said coals." This enemy of health is still used in its crude state in our towns; but it is likely that coal will cease to be thus used in another generation or two.

The smoke and effluvia of London gave point to Milton's reference in the following lines:

> As one who long in populous city pent,
> Where houses thick, and sewers annoy the air;
> Forth issuing on a summer's morn to breathe
> Among the pleasant villages and farms
> Adjoined, from each thing met conceives delight.

Kingsley (1819–1875), writing of some of the worst parts of London in the early part of the nineteenth century, was not exaggerating in the following lines:

> I turned into an alley 'neath the wall,
> And stepped from earth to hell. The light of heaven,

> The common air, was narrow, gross, and dun;
> The tiles did drop from the eaves; the unhinged doors
> Tottered over inky pools, where reeked and curdled
> The offal of a life; the gaunt-haunched swine
> Growled at their christened playmates o'er the scraps.
> Shrill mothers cursed; wan children wailed; sharp coughs
> Rang thro' the crazy chambers; hungry eyes
> Glared dumb reproach.

Similar conditions were not restricted to one country. Thus Mapother (op. cit., p. 324) quotes Dr. James of the Council of Hygiene of New York, who says:

> The dark and cheerless rear tenement, with its unventilated apartments, its damp and dingy walls, and the attendant neglect of sanitary matters, is wholly incompatible with man's social and moral nature, destroys all noble aspirations, ruins the most vigorous health, and opens wide the gate to mental, moral, physical, and spiritual death. . . . . Hence it is that the husband spends his evenings at the neighbouring dram-shop, etc.

Similarly in the report of the Massachusetts Sanitary Commission, 1850, every page of which is worth reading, and to which are attached the names of Jemuel Shattuck, N. P. Banks and Jehiel Abbott, there is a vivid description of American city conditions inimical to health, followed by the following comment: "a vast amount of unnecessarily impaired health and physical debility exists; tens of thousands of cases of preventable sickness occur; these preventable evils impose upon the people unnumbered and immeasurable calamities," etc. This report is noteworthy in the emphasis laid on the ethical side of sanitary neglect. Thus after stating that "wherever there is a dirty street, court, or dwelling house, the elements of pestilence are at work in that neighbourhood," it is pointed out that the person who permits his neighbour's atmosphere to be contaminated by filth, etc., is "worse than a highway robber. The latter robs us of property, the former of life."

It would be easy to multiply instances of endemic conditions of filth favouring disease, and some further illustrations will be found in the next chapter; but for details the special sanitary and social reports of the past and various books on social progress must be consulted.

The window tax imposed by Pitt in 1784 to raise money for the Continental wars, and not repealed until 1851, was the cause of much ill-health in the people. It was in effect an ignorant attack on fresh air and sunlight, favouring darkness and filth. Many old houses can still be seen with some of their windows bricked up to reduce this tax, a reminder of the many pits out of which we have been delivered.

Among these may be named the intra-mural burial-grounds which formerly were universal. That concentrated putrid emanations from these churchyards and churches were inimical to health is undoubted, and the abolition of town cemeteries was a great sanitary improvement. It is doubtful, however, to what extent such emanations could "impart to fevers which have arisen from other causes a typhoid or putrid character;" and still more doubtful that they "furnish the principal cause of the most developed form of typhus—that is to say, the plague." To connect plague with burials and even with burial of victims of plague, in the light of present knowledge, appears to imply the hypothesis of protracted life of the bacillus pestis in non-living matter, or the raiding of recent corpses of plague patients by rats or other rodents.

The subject of air pollution will receive consideration in the next chapter.

SOCIAL IMPROVEMENT

Although it can be little beyond an enumeration of what Simon has well named *New Momenta*, the social and moral influences making for hygienic reform call for passing notice. These factors, which in the truest sense of the word, form an intrinsic part of preventive medicine, are discussed more fully in the author's *Public Health and Insurance: American Addresses* published in 1920. Vice, especially alcoholism and sexual vice, are closely connected with disease; alcoholism is an enemy of personal and communal health in many directions and by many channels. For women and children it is a common cause of deprivation of adequate nourishment and of neglect; and any complete description of preventive medicine should lay stress on its prevention as a chief aim. Destitution from whatever cause is a progenitor of disease; and economic considerations therefore must bear an important part in the wider aspect of preventive medicine.

Personal conduct is at the back of a large share of our health or sickness, personal and that of others; and foremost among the influences bringing about the sanitary reforms of the nineteenth century must be placed the growth of a humanitarian outlook, previously lacking. In England, and to some extent in other countries, the people, including the rich, in the eighteenth and in the earlier part of the nineteenth century had a general attitude towards suffering which is in marked contrast to our present increasing humane sensitiveness. The earlier period was one of almost unmitigated industrialism, agricultural and manufacturing, and of rapid migration of population from rural districts, where altruism might act to a limited extent, to towns in which it was fortuitous, and the usual standard was unmerciful. Economic views, crystallised in the phrase *laissez faire*, *laissez aller*, were predominant and almost universal. The earlier semi-paternal control of the economic life of the people under the influence of Adam Smith, of Malthus, and of other teachers, had been replaced by inaction based on the view that any interference with freedom of competition in obtaining work or in employing workers is useless or mischievous.

This rigid doctrine was challenged by men who were imbued with the motives of humanitarianism and most of whom were influenced by evangelical Christianity. The Wesleyan movement, led by John

Wesley (1703–1791) had enormous influence in bringing about an increasing rebellion against this exclusively economic outlook. John Howard (1726–1790), in his historical work of prison reform, was largely influenced by these motives, as were also William Wilberforce (1759–1833) and his associates in their work for the abolition of the slave-trade in the West Indies, crowned with victory in 1807.

The movement for reduction of the cruelty involved in the protracted duration of work in factories and mines and in the conditions of this work, particularly as regards children and women, was activated also by evangelistic and humanitarian ideals, although it may be agreed that the rival politics of the land interest and of the manufacturing rich played a part.

Sanitary and poor-law reform were being actively advocated in the same period, and these reforms as well as the agitation for diminution of the cruelty implied in insanitary homes and in the savage conditions of industry, were witness to the wave of improvement in the national conscience, which was manifesting itself in these and in other departments of human life.

Even more strikingly than in unreformed factory and mining conditions and in the fever-infested slums of our cities, the low value attached to life and the cruelty in its wastage was shown in the enforcement of capital punishment for some 160 different offenses, including at one time theft of an article of the value of more than one shilling. It was only in

1861 that punishment by death was limited to treason and wilful murder; and prior to Peel's Acts, 1824–1829, many financial frauds were punishable by hanging. This ferocity of punishment showed also a lack of vision of the possibility of preventing crime, by an adequate police force, rendering the detection of crime easy, and its punishment proportioned to the crime; and thus making judge and juries willing to convict the guilty. So likewise with other punishments. The pillory was virtually abolished in 1816; public flogging was made illegal in 1817, and in 1820 a further Act prohibited the private flogging of female offenders.

The growth of humanitarian ideals spread gradually to every branch of social and industrial life. It captured bit by bit the legislature, it overwhelmed the inertia of those who should have been leaders in reform, it gradually put to blush and exposed to the rack of publicity the exploiters of oppressed labour, the landlords of insanitary dwellings, the local authorities who were neglecting their elementary duties to the poor and for the prevention of epidemics, and the many others whose vested interests were delaying reform. The triumph of higher ideals is far from complete at the present day, but a comparison with the past gives hope and confidence for the future.

Indeed much of our progress in public health owed its initiation and its driving power to the cultivation of Mercy, to the increasing sensitiveness of the public conscience which has made suffering which is avoidable increasingly repugnant to the national sentiment. The general movement towards mercy spread over into animal life, which is an additional reason why public health workers should interest themselves in every movement for the mitigation or avoidance of animal suffering.

To deal with cruelty to animals by legal enactment involved a new principle of legislation for criminal law. It extended the protection of the weak against the strong beyond human relationships to the relationship between man and his living animal property. In view of this, the first British enactment with this object, which was passed in 1822, and which is commonly known as "Martin's Act," may be regarded as an epochal date in the history of the control of cruelty to animals.

This Act, which has been amended and extended many times since its enactment, included provisions against the starving of impounded animals, and for the regulation of slaughter-houses.

CHAPTER XIII

Progress in the Eighteenth and Early Part of the Nineteenth Century

Resuming the story already begun in Chapters VII and subsequent chapters we must now attempt to indicate the slow progress towards the light in the one hundred fifty to two hundred years preceding what may be called the Pasteurian period. This progress was on several lines: a differentiation of diseases one from another; an increasing realisation of the part played by overcrowding and dirt, whether of respiratory or excremental origin, in the production of communicable diseases; and varying efforts to prevent the spread of infection. The differentiation between typhus and typhoid fever came late; and before these two had been generally recognised as separate diseases some of the work needed for the rapid reduction of one of them (typhus fever) had already been accomplished. It may be added here that the disappearance of typhus long before the microörganism causing it had been discovered and before the louse had been ascertained to be its vector, is one of the most striking events in epidemiology. Of equal interest is the disappearance of Plague from most countries, before it had become known that this disease is spread by fleas passing from specifically infected rats to man. In both instances it happened that efforts directed blindly against filth and overcrowding had incidentally diminished the possibilities of infection. The clearing of slums, the limewashing of infected rooms, the cleansing of their contents, the segregation of the sick in "fever" hospitals in the one case: and, in the other case, improved sanitation, diminishing the readiness of access of rats into dwellings, along with the replacement of the black by the brown rat (page 82) had reduced the channels of infection, and in innumerable instances broken the link between case and case.

In typhoid fever and its congeners a similar story can be told. Excremental contamination sooner or later meant specific conveyance of typhoid germs; and steady improvement in regard to closets, drains and sewers, and especially in preventing the contamination of drinking water and milk had greatly diminished the mortality from typhoid fever before the Eberth bacillus was recognised. But, although history reveals the above course of events, it is none the less true that the discovery that, in plague, infection is spread solely, except in pneumonic plague, by the bites of fleas infected by rats or other rodents with the Bacillus pestis; that in typhus fever, there is no fear of infection apart from lice acquired from a typhus patient; and that in typhoid fever, specific infection alone causes the disease; and that, furthermore, the presence of this infection can be determined by laboratory tests, has rendered possible more exact measures of prevention, and has enabled the practitioner in preventive medicine to promote sanitary measures with an economy and directness of effort not previously attainable.

After this preliminary statement, we may now indicate some of the stages of progress in the period named at the head of this chapter.

Much light is thrown on the subject by Sir John Pringle's *Observations on the Diseases of the British Army*, first published in 1752. Pringle may be said to be the father of military medicine; and he and Lind (pages 106 and 194) were forerunners of the early public health reforms. Pringle's work is chiefly concerned with descriptions of the incidence of disease among troops in Flanders. Here we can indicate only his views on infectious diseases. Referring to jail or hospital fever he advanced certain conjectures, though he was alive to the fact that "we too often see the judgment influenced and perverted by such speculations." He attached importance to the "septic principle," and he was encouraged to prosecute this subject, first because of the large number of "putrid cases" that were under his care in hospitals abroad, and secondly in view of Lord Verulam's (Bacon's) authority, who "offers good reasons for considering the knowledge of what brings on, and what retards putrefaction, as most likely to account for some of the more abstruse operations of nature." Pringle regarded "putrefaction of the air, as being of all the causes of sickness perhaps the most fatal and the least understood." He classified the bad air hurtful to an army as of four kinds: (a) arising from the corrupted air of marshes; (b) from human excrements lying about the camp in hot weather, when the dysentery is frequent; (c) from straw rotting in the tents; (d) that which is "breathed in hospitals crowded with men ill of putrid distempers." The last named form of bad air may arise also in dirty thickly populated barracks, and in crowded transport ships on long voyages. In all these forms of bad air, the miasma of putrid effluvia was regarded as the main factor; but "when they contained the putrid excrements and effluvia of the sick, they are then more infectious and dangerous." In regard to dysentery, Pringle is definite as to infection, saying "the great source of infection seems to be the privies, after they have received the dysenteric excrements of those who first fall ill."

Pringle identified hospital fever with the jail-distemper, (typhus fever), but although he attached some importance to "pestilential infection," it is not clear that by this he meant transmission from a typhus patient; and he avers that he has known instances of this fever "beginning in a ward, where there was no other cause but one of the men having a mortified limb." He also held the view that a person suffering from a putrid disease, such as smallpox or dysentery, who lies in a small and close apartment "may fall into this malignant fever." Pringle's practice was as sound as was possible in the then state of knowledge. He laid stress on the importance of fresh air, on dryness and warmth for the soldiers, on the need for frequently changing camp, and on small regimental hospitals, rather than crowding into larger general hospitals.

He recommended the apparatus proposed by Dr. Stephen Hales, a great pioneer in ventilation, for introduction in all sick rooms. This was a sort of double bellows, for alternate exhaustion and propulsion of air.

As the growth of Army sanitation in the last hundred years cannot be separately discussed, it is convenient to add here that civilian hygiene has occasionally been first initiated in the Army, where the conditions of military discipline enable fairly exact results to be obtained. Undoubtedly the greatest gain in Army hygiene has resulted from the introduction of antiseptic treatment of wounds. Next to this probably should be put the recent chlorination of all drinking waters in temperate countries, and the protection of soldiers against mosquitoes in tropical countries. Anti-typhoid inoculation has had marked influence in decreasing typhoid infections, where satisfactory sanitation was impracticable. During the Boer War (1899–1900), disease, especially dysentery and typhoid fever, were a more serious cause of loss of life and of efficient service than the casualties of fighting. In the Great War, 1914–1918, this had ceased to hold, and excepting trench fever (a newly recognised clinical entity, spread by lice) and venereal disease, sickness was remarkably small in amount.

Sanitary progress owes much to laymen without special scientific knowledge. In England Edwin Chadwick, Lord Shaftesbury, Florence Nightingale and some others have been among the earliest to realise the possibilities of preventive medicine; and in the United States the names of Lemuel Shattuck, a layman, and of his colleagues (page 94) deserve to be held in remembrance.

But before the activities of these early missionaries of pity and health could have any prospect of success, individual and some degree of communal effort had been elicited in a number of centres, sometimes by physicians and notably in one instance by a prince of reformers, John Howard, who was not a doctor. This movement can be illustrated by reference to Chester, to Manchester and to Liverpool, as well as to Howard's own work and to the work which was being done for the Army and Navy by Pringle and Lind and their contemporaries. The efforts thus exemplified were a necessary preliminary to the later work of Southwood Smith and Edwin Chadwick. In studying the more generally known work of the sanitary period, from 1830 onwards, one must not overlook its anticipations in this earlier period.

James Lind (1716–1794) had shewn that in naval hospitals, often containing patients impressed from the prisons, jail fever (typhus) did not spread beyond a narrow area around the patient's bed. He also shewed that the infective agent is carried in filthy garments, and urged destruction of their infection by great heat, such as that of an oven. In 1781 arrangements were made for receiving newly impressed men on board "slop ships," where they were cleansed and supplied with new clothing, before going to their ships. By this means much typhus was prevented. Dr. John Haygarth of Chester opened fever wards in the infirmary at Chester in 1784, in which Lind's rules were first applied to hospital treatment in civilian practice. The rules for work in these wards are given on page 209 of John Howard's *An Account of the principal Lazarettos in Europe*, 2nd edition, 1791, and comprised the following among other items: no communication of patients or nurses with other parts of the house; provision of clean linen for patients; frequent washing of floors; all foul linen to be placed at once in water and to be washed out twice in clean water; all windows in the ward to be kept constantly open; etc.

Attached to the above-mentioned work is a letter dated May 1789, written by Haygarth, which gives some further particulars of his enlightened views. He states that he has "long thought that perfect purification from pestilential contagion might be performed with great ease and certainty." He advocates "the completest perflation of air" for hospitals. Referring to his Chester experience, he clearly enunciates the main object of fever hospitals.

> The chief aim of our regulations is not merely to preserve the lives of infected persons. The principal purpose

and benefit of the establishment is to prevent any infectious fever from spreading through poor families, and through the town.

And he refers in sanguine terms to "the success of our small-pox society, in checking the progress of the variolous contagion, in closely adjoining houses" by similar measures.

In Manchester a "House of Recovery" was opened in 1796, with similar managements to the fever ward of Chester Infirmary, and Dr. John Ferriar (*Medical Histories and Reflections*, 4 vols., 1810–1813), writing about a similar House erected in Stockport, said "I believe there is not a town in the Kingdom containing four thousand inhabitants which would not be greatly benefited by similar establishments."

In 1795, largely owing to the advocacy of Percival, assisted by Ferriar, a voluntary Board of Health was formed in Manchester, which received influential support. Rewards were given to those reporting cases of fever, washing and cleansing were advocated, as well as segregation of the sick in the House of Recovery. In Liverpool Dr. Currie, was advocating similar measures; and in 1801 a House of Recovery was opened in that city, which was supported out of parish rates. In 1833, Dr. Duncan, giving evidence as to the utility of this institution, stated that while previous to its opening cases of typhus fever formed one-fourth of all the poor-law cases, they did not in that year exceed one-tenth or one-twelfth. Other towns, including London, followed these examples;

and in assessing the value of the various measures taken against typhus, hospital segregation must be given a high place.

A foremost position as a pioneer in sanitary reform must be accorded to John Howard (1726–1790), whose work led to the abolition from prisons of typhus fever (jail distemper), which on many occasions had infected judge and jury called on to try prisoners coming from infected cells. The story of his work is well known; he was the first systematically to use two of our chief modern means of ascertaining evils, viz., inspections to ascertain the exact circumstances and conditions, and reporting with statistical summaries of ascertained facts. It is on such data that action must be based, and it is by such summarised statements that the need for further powers of action can be brought home to those in authority. The conditions in some of the prisons visited by him were so vile that "the leaves of my memorandum book were often so tainted that I could not use it till after spreading it an hour or two before the fire." . . . . "From my own observations in 1773, 1774 and 1775 I was fully convinced that many more prisoners were destroyed by the gaol fever than were put to death by all the public executions in the Kingdom." Howard had no doubt as to the spread of infection from person to person.

It is noteworthy that fifty years later typhus fever was unknown in British prisons; but it continued outside these prisons, due to the contagion which in prisons had been prevented by reform. Further illustrations bearing on the prevention of typhus fever, and its relation to extreme poverty, will be found in Chapter XV; and the efforts of Lind and Blane to eradicate scurvy from the British Navy, with the contemporaneous work of Captain Cook are further noted in Chapter XXI.

HEALTH OF THE COMMUNITY AS A SOCIAL CONCERN

In the last chapter mention has been made of the advance of altruism, the rapid increase in moral sensitiveness, which was associated with and largely due to the Wesleyan revival. This began about the year 1738; and as Simon has put it "from the middle of the century onward, the evangelical revival carried among its chief consequences, that man learnt to feel new solicitudes for man; and under the new influence, new associations were extensively organised for dealing with the various sorts of social evil" (page 132, *English Sanitary Institutions*). Much importance attaches also to the influences implied in two great historical events, namely the Declaration of American Independence of 1776, and the French Revolution beginning in 1789–1790, which like the impetus originating from religious enthusiasm opened the way towards good government for the well-being of the common people.

Under these influences there was an increasing departure from the policy which Thomas Carlyle loved to call securing "strength for the strong, want for the weak, and devil take the hindmost." Efforts having reform in view, whether concerned with reduced hours of industrial work, sanitation, improved housing, or the safeguarding of food supplies, were regarded by many serious people as the obvious beginning of socialism; and hard work, on the part of many reformers was needed to drive the plough of reform through the stiff clay of prejudice. Here we are concerned with the science of preventive medicine and with the motives which led to its practice, not with an account of this practice; and from this standpoint it will suffice to set out the following dates without further attempt to dilate upon their social significance.

1738—Beginning of the Methodist revival.

1774—John Howard testified to the House of Commons on his famous visitation of prisons.

1781—Robert Raikes began his Sunday Schools.

1769–1785—Granville Sharp, Ramsay and Clarkson wrote against the toleration of slavery.

1784—Fever wards opened at Chester.

1788–1789—Wilberforce was supported in House of Commons by Pitt, Fox and Burke in proposing resolutions for the abolition of the Slave Trade.

1807—Abolition Bill passed forbidding trading in slaves.

1833—Holding of slaves in British dominions forbidden, and 20 millions sterling voted for compensation to owners of slaves.

1808–1818—Romilly's successive reforms for humanising the criminal law.

1822—First enactment against cruelty to animals.

1825—Repeal of enactments making it unlawful for workmen to take combined action.
1832—Health and Morals Act to regulate the Labour of Bound Children in Cotton Factories.
1834—Poor Law Amendment Act.
1835—Municipal Corporations Act.
1836—Registration of Births, Marriages and Deaths Act.

It is not intended in this volume to deal with the Parliamentary enactments which gradually made preventive medicine increasingly operative; but the above dates, and some others which will be given in later pages are placed on record as indicating progress in appreciation of the practice of altruism, on which the application of preventive medicine in public health administration, in large measure depends.

In the next chapter, the relation of several important pioneers in public health to the progress in preventive medicine is considered. The illustrations given are chiefly of British experience; as the teachings of preventive medicine were applied in Britain at an earlier period than in other countries.

CHAPTER XIV

Poverty and Preventive Medicine

Stress has been laid in preceding chapters on the influence of increasing sensitiveness to human suffering and desire to alleviate or prevent it as a motive in sanitary reform. But there were two other motives which also had profound weight, viz. fear and economic motives. Panic was a large factor in securing repentance and good works when cholera threatened; as it, likewise, was in an earlier century when plague became epidemic; and in both instances the desire for complete and accurate information as to the extent of the invasion led in England to the call for accurate vital statistics. It may truly be said that the early adoption of accurate registration of births and deaths was hastened by fears of cholera, and by the intelligent realisation that one must know the localisation as well as the number of the enemy to be fought.

The first Parish Registers of Death were kept in England in 1538; and the "Bills of Mortality" for London were published towards the end of the same century, in order to quiet public fears by giving a correct account of the progress of the plague.

At intervals attempts were made to extend this registration. In 1665 Captain John Graunt had published a valuable analysis of the Bills of Mortality, in which their value and defects were discussed. In 1754 Dr. John Fothergill (*Life*, by Dr. R. Hingston Fox, 1919) in a petition to the Company of Parish Clerks in London set forth the defects of the weekly Bills and the injudicious character of the list of diseases, and proposed that all the parishes in England should be obliged to keep registers of births, burials and marriages; that county registers should be compiled, and these made the subject in the capital of a general Bill or Summary. The Company applied to Parliament for powers to carry these proposals into effect, but the inclusion of a clause for numbering the people led to the defeat of the proposals. There was clamorous reference to the "sin of David," and it was not until 1801 that the first national census was secured. National registration of deaths etc. did not begin until 1836. Reference should be made also to Dr. Thos. Percival's "Proposals for establishing more Accurate and Comprehensive Bills of Mortality" (published in his *Essays Medical and Experimental*, London, 1773, Vol. I). He prefixed his essay on this subject with the appropriate motto from Ovid: "Fas est et ab hoste doceri," and set out with much learning and foresight the great national advantages which since then have been obtained from 1836 onward. Like Farr at a later period he sensed the immense social and hygienic value of accurate vital statistics; and Percival's essay gives a remarkably acute foresight of what Farr was in later years privileged to accomplish. In Sweden the parish registration of births, marriages, and deaths had been made compulsory in 1686.

In 1831–1832 nearly 42,000 deaths were caused by cholera in Great Britain and Ireland; and during 1831 Local Boards of Health were formed voluntarily in many parts of the country. These made spasmodic and imperfect efforts to sweep the Augean stables of insalubriousness. The need for a complete registration of deaths became evident, and, the necessary enactments having been passed, the office of Registrar General of Births, Deaths and Marriages in England was created in 1836; and the appointment of Dr. William Farr as statistical expert to this office was followed by the issue of a series of reports which have guided sanitary reform and incited it year by year to increased activity.

Later on the need for corresponding returns of sickness caused by infectious disease became evident, and the compulsory notification of such diseases by doctors has been an important factor in enabling early measures of isolation and disinfection to be taken, in linking up infectious cases with one another, and in thus tracing their source. Benjamin Ward Richardson, writing of Farr's reports—and the remark is even truer of our present position—said it is no longer true that pestilence walketh in the dark. It is measured and registered, walketh at last in the open day.

The economic motive as well as the motive of panic was concerned in the promotion of accurate and complete vital statistics; and as leader in the English campaign for economising on sickness, Edwin Chadwick (1800–1890) must be given the first place. He was foremost as a promoter of preventive medicine, with an urgent desire for its immediate application.

Edwin Chadwick, was educated for the bar; and in his early years wrote largely for journals. In 1828 he wrote an article on Life Insurance for the *Westminster Review*, which probably determined his future career. It dealt with the expectation of life and the influence of environment upon it. His writing attracted the attention of Jeremy Bentham, with whom Chadwick became intimate, and there is little doubt that Bentham's advice and his utilitarian philosophy largely influenced Chadwick's life. In 1832 Chadwick was appointed an Assistant Commissioner to inquire into the working of the Poor Laws, soon after the meeting of the Reform Act Parliament of that year. This was a period of active reform. Within three or four years of this time paid police came into being, the inspection of factories began, and municipal politics were reformed. In 1833 a Factory Commission was appointed to inquire into the shocking condition of children employed in the Cotton trade. One member of this small Commission of three was Dr. Southwood Smith, and Chadwick was its secretary. Although it is not intended in this volume to enter into details of administration, it is relevant to note that the most important recommendation of this Commission was in favour of the appointment of professional paid inspectors to supervise the carrying out of the factory regulations. The need for inspection as a means of reform had been demonstrated by Howard for prisons. The introduction of paid professional inspectors of factories, not subject to local influences, and standing in an impartial position between the employer and the employed, represented an extremely important advance in the practice of preventive medicine, which has gradually been extended to all branches of public health and social work. The employment of such paid inspectors was the beginning of the end of inertia in factory reform; and this reform was followed very shortly by a recommendation of the Poor Law Commission for the appointment of paid relieving officers as permanent officials to undertake the giving of relief on a uniform scale. So much it is desirable to state in these pages—which are concerned primarily with causes and principles, not with administration—; for the subsequent administrative course of public health administration centers round the work of paid inspectors, whether they are known under the name of medical officers of health, sanitary inspectors, or health visitors.

Turning to the second motive for public health progress noted above, i.e., economic considerations, it is necessary to indicate briefly the way in which in England the science of preventive medicine and public health originated in large measure in the work of the Poor Law organization. Down to 1834 the organization of poor relief was a purely parochial affair; and between 1782 and 1834 the parish officers who administered this relief in many parts of the country had made their allowances work out as a recognized means of supplementing wages. This was demoralizing to all concerned; for in practice it meant, for instance, that farmers agreed to pay their workers, say, a shilling a day, leaving the ratepayers as a whole to pay another shilling, in order that the labourer and his family might live.

Chadwick and his colleagues recommended drastic reforms, including a large measure of control of local administration by a central authority, and the Poor Law Act of 1834 aimed at organizing poor relief on a uniform basis. With the degree of success which was attained we are not concerned; but it is fairly clear that the Poor Law Commission, whose Secretary was Chadwick, had not yet fully grasped the idea that the causes of poverty, which lead to pauperism, must wherever possible be attacked. But facing the storm of opposition which the Poor Law Board aroused, Chadwick by means of frequent investigations soon realised that a large share of total pauperism was due to the miserable housing and sanitation of the poor, as well as to overwork in various occupations; and the Factory Act of 1833, with its institution of factory inspectors, and the establishment of national registration of deaths, in both of which reforms Chadwick was largely concerned, were the first fruits of reform leading to public health progress. The great cholera epidemic of 1831 also may be described as among the chief hasteners of reform.

In 1839 the Poor Law Commissioners wrote a letter to the then Home Secretary, Lord John Russell, which shews their appreciation of the relation of insanitation and sickness to pauperism:

> The most prominent and pressing of the first class of charges for which provision appears to be required are for the means of averting the charges upon the poor rates which are caused by nuisances by which contagion is generated and persons are reduced to destitution. . . . Labourers are suddenly thrown by infectious disease into a state of destitution for which immediate relief must be given. In the case of death the widow and children are thrown as paupers on the parish.

The letter than urges the need for applying to the legislature "for immediate measures for the removal of these constantly-acting causes of destitution and death."

The progress of administrative reforms is traced in outline in my book on *The Ministry of Health*, 1925 (G. P. Putnams), and it is not proposed to follow it further in these pages; but the above extract shews a full realization of the important fact, that a large share of the total national destitution could be avoided by preventing preventable pestilences.

Striking statistics were given by Southwood Smith in his *Report on the Physical Causes of Sickness and Mortality, to which the Poor are particularly exposed, and which are capable of Prevention by Sanitary Measures*, 1837. In the preceding year more than one-fifth of the total recipients of relief in London were the subjects of fever. The proportion in Bethnal Green was one-third, in Whitechapel one-half, and in the parish of St. George-the-Martyr, was as much as 87 per cent of the total recipients of relief.[1]

[1] On the subject of this and several other chapters, fuller information is contained in *The Nation's Health: A Review of the Works of Edwin Chadwick*, edited by B. Ward Richardson (2 vols. Longmans 1887), and in *The Public Health Agitation*, 1838–1848 by B. L. Hutchins (Fifield, 1909); and in *Health, Wealth and Population in the Early Days of the Industrial Revolution* by M. C. Buer, B.Sc. (Rontledge, 1926), published when this volume was going to press.

CHAPTER XV

The Prevention of "Fever"

The dependence of a large part of the total misery and destitution in the community on the "fever" which was endemic in crowded centres being realised, the means for diminishing "fever" came more and more under consideration. The same means were assumed to be equally successful against cholera, to which a separate chapter will be devoted.

Dr. Southwood Smith, and other physicians, among whom should be specially mentioned Drs. Arnott and Kaye, were employed by the Poor Law Board to investigate and advise. They made surveys of the sanitary conditions in London and a number of provincial towns, and inquired into the incidence of "fever" in different localities. Dr. Southwood Smith has left behind him various writings from which one can obtain an accurate idea of the conceptions of preventive medicine at this period which were so fruitful in successful reform.

Born in 1788, Southwood Smith lived until 1861, and crowded into the official period of his life (1833–1854) a vast amount of beneficent work. His views were accepted by Chadwick and formed the propulsive power of Chadwick's masterful work.

Southwood Smith's essential teaching was that there was an intrinsic connection between epidemics and local insanitary conditions. When he began his work personal infection was regarded as supremely important. Thus in the first outbreak of Asiatic Cholera in 1831, the Royal College of Physicians gave the following opinion, which was published throughout the land in the form of an Order of the King in Council. They first of all endorsed Mead's views as to the efficacy of quarantine (page 81) and expressed the view that "measures of external precaution for preventing the introduction of the cholera morbus by a rigorous quarantine have hitherto been found effectual," and they then gave the following official recommendations:

> To carry into effect the separation of the sick from the healthy, it would be very expedient that one or more houses should be kept in view in each town or its neighbourhood, as places to which every case of the disease, as soon as detected, might be removed, provided the family of the afflicted person consent to such removal; and, in case of refusal, a conspicuous mark, "*Sick*," should be placed in front of the house, to warn persons that it is in quarantine; and even when persons with the disease shall have been removed, and the house shall have been purified, the word "*Caution*" should be substituted, as denoting suspicion of the disease; and the inhabitants of such house should not be at liberty to move out or communicate with other persons until, by the authority of the local board, the mark shall have been removed.
>
> It is recommended that those who may fall victims to this most formidable disease should be buried in a detached ground, in the vicinity of the house that may have been selected for the reception of cholera patients. By this regulation, it is intended to confine, as much as possible, every source of infec-

tion to one spot; on the same principle, all persons who may be employed in the removal of the sick from their own houses, as well as all who may attend upon cholera patients in the capacity of nurses, should live apart from the rest of the community.

Whenever objections arise to the removal of the sick from the healthy, or other causes exist to render such a step not advisable, the same prospect of success in extinguishing the seeds of the pestilence cannot be expected. Much, however, may be done, even in these difficult circumstances, by following the same principles of prudence, and by avoiding all unnecessary communication with the public out of doors: all articles of food or other necessaries required by the family should be placed in front of the house, and received by one of the inhabitants of the house after the person delivering them shall have retired. Until the time during which the contagion of cholera lies dormant in the human frame has been more minutely ascertained, it will be necessary, for the sake of perfect security, that convalescents from the disease, and those who have had any communication with them, should be kept under observation for a period of not less than twenty days.

All intercourse with any infected town and the neighbouring country must be prevented, by the best means within the power of the magistrates, who will have to make regulations for the supply of provisions.

Other measures of a more coercive nature may be rendered expedient for the common safety, if unfortunately so fatal a disease should ever show itself in this country, in the terrific way in which it has appeared in various parts of Europe; and it may become necessary to draw troops or a strong body of police around infected places, so as utterly to exclude the inhabitants from all intercourse with the country: and we feel sure that what is demanded for the common safety of the state, will always be acquiesced in with a willing submission to the necessity which imposes it.

In emphasizing the limitations of the utility of quarantine Southwood Smith set himself against the teaching of the above memorandum, which was described as "the dogmatism of the lecture-room;" and his six years' work from 1824 onwards as physician to the London Fever Hospital, backed by daily visits to the dwellings of dispensary patients led him to the conclusions:

1. That epidemics break out and spread in districts of limited extent having uniformly some sanitary defects.

2. That the extension and spread of these diseases are very exactly proportioned to the extent of bad sanitary conditions, disappearing as soon as these conditions are amended, and never appearing where they are good.

3. That epidemics are preventable, since their development and spread are dependent on definite conditions, invariably existing in infected localities, and which it is in our power to remedy.

4. That epidemics are not necessarily diseases of poverty; the susceptibility to them being created by want—not of food—but of pure air; and such diseases being chiefly prevalent among the poor, because it is their unhappy lot to live in the worst sanitary districts, and because the air in and around their dwellings is for the most part poisoned by filth.

5. That fever is pre-eminently the disease of adult age, being nearly four times more prevalent between the ages of 20 and 30 than it is under 20 or between 30 and 40, and fourteen times more prevalent between 20 and 30 than between 40 and 60.

Two conclusions of the utmost importance necessarily resulted from the perhaps unduly generalised statements given above. They are given in Southwood Smith's own words:

1. That fever is the great pauperizer of the country, because it attacks the working classes precisely during the ten years when they have the greatest number of young children dependent on them for support; because it destroys the heads of families, depriving the wife of her husband and the children of their parents at the very age when such children are most helpless.

2. That fever and other epidemics are preventable diseases, since, as has been stated, their existence depends on certain definite, palpable, and uniform conditions invariably present in epidemic districts, but which are under the control of man.

In two important official reports to the Poor Law Commissioners (1837–1838) Southwood Smith placed special emphasis on what he termed the *localizing causes* of disease, these being "the conditions on which the outbreak and development of epidemics invariably and everywhere depend," and the general purport of his teaching is further displayed in the following extracts from two lectures given by him at the Philosophical Institution, Edinburgh, November, 1855.

The whole tenour of experience shews that whatever produces an especial liability to one epidemic, produces a similar liability to every other.

The pre-disposing causes of epidemics are:

1. External, which vitiate the air.

2. Internal, which more immediately vitiate the blood.

Besides the contamination of the air by external causes, the air itself undergoes natural changes which pre-dispose it to the development and spread of epidemics.

Strictly speaking, however, all that we really know is this—that where certain conditions exist, epidemics break out and spread; that where those conditions do not exist, epidemics do not break out and spread; and that where those conditions did exist, but have been removed, thereupon epidemics cease to break out and spread.

After discussing the existence of some special agent producing each disease, Southwood Smith concluded as follows:

> One thing is certain, that practically our concern is with the known causes—the ascertained conditions. These are palpable, definite, and capable of complete removal and prevention. Overcrowding, for example, we can prevent; the accumulation of filth in towns and houses we can prevent; the supply of light, air, and water, together with the several other appliances included in the all-comprehensive word *Cleanliness*, we can secure. To the extent to which it is in our power to do this, it is in our power to prevent epidemics.

In holding these views, it will be clear from the perusal of preceding chapters that Southwood Smith was inbued with the conception of *miasma*, which has run right through the ages. If text books of medicine, e.g., Ziemssen's Cyclopedia of the Practice of Medicine, of so recent a date as 1875, are consulted, it will be seen that infectious diseases were still divided into *miasmatic* and *contagious*. In this classification, miasm is used in contradistinction to contagium, but older writers speak of the miasm of measles or smallpox; and with them personal infection played a relatively insignificant part if it was admitted at all. The doctrine prevalent when the sanitary renaissance began in England,—as shewn by the preceding extracts from Southwood Smith—was that while malaria was due to some virus generated de novo in marshy districts, "fever" and even cholera might similarly be engendered in circumstances of organic filth and overcrowding without the participation in their causation of a preceding case. To explain the absence or lesser prevalence of these diseases in non-epidemic intervals, there was needed the conception of an "epidemic constitution," a phrase employed by Sydenham, though the conception dates back to Hippocrates. There were differences of opinion as to the nature of the virus causing "fever" or cholera when thus developed or created. These differences are indicated in the extracts given on pages 135–136. They are further exemplified in the following extract from Bristowe's *Treatise on the Theory and Practice of Medicine*, second edition, 1878.

> Dr. Murchison argues forcibly in favour of its origin (i.e., of the specific poison of enteric fever) independently of the disease which it generates. Dr. Budd and others argue with equal vehemence in support of the opposite hypothesis. We incline strongly to the latter view, and in accordance with it, are disposed at present to regard the essential cause of enteric fever not as a mere inorganic or even organic result of decomposition, but like other contagia, as an organised living particle which has special endowments and unlimited powers of multiplication.

At this point it is desirable to define "fever." As used in the early period of sanitary reform, it included typhus fever, typhoid or enteric fever, the varieties of paratyphoid infection, and probably also relapsing or famine fever. There is little doubt also that owing to lack of knowledge of the natural history of each disease or lack of medical skill, cerebro-spinal fever, acute tuberculosis, and some other diseases were sometimes inadequately diagnosed as "fever." The two chief constituents of the term were doubtless typhus and typhoid fever. The national registration returns did not distinguish these two prior to 1869. For convenience of reference the historical course of the mortality registered from the two chief diseases included in the term "fever" is shewn in the following table.

England and Wales. Death-rates per million persons

	1851–1860	1861–1870	1871–1880	1881–1890	1891–1900	1901–1910	1911–1920
"Fever"	908	885	482	235	183	94	
Typhus			57	14	3	1	*
Enteric			332	198	174	91	35

* Typhus fever has almost disappeared. In the eleven years 1915–1925 it caused 28 deaths.

Until the differentiation of typhus and enteric fever was made, it is evident that an exact study of the circumstances in which each arises was impossible, unless—contrary to the facts—it were assumed that they have a causation in common, the difference between their clinical features being determined by collateral atmospheric or other external conditions. This view at one time was almost universal. Hence in the history of preventive medicine importance attaches to the differentiation of these two diseases.

As is well known, in death from enteric fever characteristic intestinal ulceration is found, this being consistently absent in typhus fever. Many earlier observers had found intestinal ulcers in certain fatal cases of "fever," and Bretonneau of Tours first proved that these ulcers were always localised in the solitary and agminated glands of the ileum (Murchison, *Continued Fevers*, third edition, 1884, page 426). Louis, Bretonneau and Chomel all inclined to the view that typhus and typhoid were identical, though deploring the absence of careful autopsies in typhus cases. Many observers recorded the differences between the two types of disease; but Murchison authoritatively states that "to Drs. Gerhard and Pennock" (who after studying under Louis in Paris had observed an epidemic of typhus in Philadelphia in in 1837) certainly belongs the credit of first establishing the most important points of distinction between typhus and enteric fevers." Dr. A. P. Stewart in Edinburgh very shortly afterwards described more accurately than had previously been done the differences between the two diseases, and emphasised the view that while enteric might occur in the best aired houses, typhus was generated from the effluvia of persons living in close and unventilated rooms. Doubt still lingered in many minds as to the distinctiveness of the two diseases; but this was removed by Sir William Jenner's researches published between 1849 and 1851.

CHAPTER XVI

The Prevention of "Fever" (continued).

Running through several preceding chapters will have been seen the struggle ever proceeding as to the genesis and means of preventing infectious diseases. And at the back of this groping and struggling, there have occurred, in ebb and flow, variations in doctrine, which may be embodied in three or four main questions.

Are we the victims of external influences, cosmic, telluric, or other, and therefore helpless to prevent or mitigate pestilences, which must wear themselves out in accordance with their unknown nature?

Are infectious diseases due always to some miasma, developed by putrefaction of vegetable matter (malaria) or of animal excreta (cholera and typhoid) or derived from the exhalations of crowded humanity (typhus fever); or from some combined effect of miasma and infection?

Are communicable diseases, never conveyed except by infection from man to man, or from animal to man? Or may they be generated *de novo* from putrefying or other matter? The gradual process of enlightenment on the above points is the subject of these chapters.

The history of Typhus Fever is the history of human misery. Its universal association in origin with destitution and dirt is undoubted. In an address to the Epidemiological Section of the Royal Society of Medicine in October, 1907, I traced this association in Ireland. Famines occurred at intervals, and there being no adequate poor-relief, the immediate effect was widespread migration of population and vagrancy, the vagrants carrying typhus fever with them in their wanderings. Similarly Irish labourers in their yearly visits to England for harvesting work scattered typhus, and Irish emigrants to the United States did likewise. The case of Typhus in Ireland is historically important; for typhus rapidly decreased when poor-relief arrangements were altered, and relief was made available in each area. By this means a large mass of previously ambulatory infection was immobilised, and the curve of the national death-rate from typhus soon shewed the effect of this indirect but effective measure in preventing the spread of infection.

But immobilization of ambulant cases of typhus in their own locality and of some of the recognised cases in general institutions, although it served to lower the incidence of the disease, could not secure its abolition; and in England, for the better care of the sick, but incidentally to diminish facilities for the spread of disease, there grew up the system of Fever Hospitals. These when first instituted were literally for "fever," i.e., for undifferentiated cases of typhoid and typhus; and a main qualification of a nurse in those days was that she had been "salted," i.e., had already had an attack of typhus. This movement started in the latter part of the eighteenth century, the first fever hospital being opened at Chester (page 107). By the middle of the nineteenth century it was generally agreed that typhus could not, with safety to others, be treated in the wards of general hospitals.

The statistics given in Murchison's Continued Fevers give a faint clue to the extent to which hospital segregation of cases was practised. Of typhus 1,070 cases were admitted into the London Fever Hospital in 1848–1850, 2,782 cases in 1851–1860, and 14,676 in 1861–1870; the number of enteric admissions in the same periods being 427, 1,845, and 3,716. The death rate in London from these two diseases and from whatever other deaths were then included under the name "Fever," varied but little until 1870, but declined from 904 per million living in 1861–1870 to 374 in 1871–1880. The increasing use of linen and still more of cotton underclothing, the clearance of slums, the regulation of lodging houses, the growing activity of sanitary authorities in limewashing infected bedrooms and in cleansing bedding etc., also played their part in reducing the prevalence of typhus fever: eventually the links of infection were entirely severed, and at the present time typhus has disappeared except as an occasional imported visitor. Ireland still serves as a rapidly decreasing reservoir of infection; and cases are introduced into England from Eastern Europe. We now know that it is spread by lice which pass directly from the sick to the healthy, or by bedding, bedclothes, or garments which have been in contact with infected persons; and that although overcrowding and dirt greatly increase the risk of infection, they do so by favouring infestation by lice; and it is not the least romantic aspect of the disappearance of typhus fever that, in western civilized countries this disease became practically extinct before it was ascertained that the louse was responsible for spreading it. No more eloquent testimony to the value of personal cleanliness, irrespective of disease, could be adduced. The recent military experience of Trench fever is in point.

The history of Enteric or Typhoid Fever is one of improvement almost as dramatic as that shown in western experience of Typhus. How has this been brought about? Since 1869 the course of this disease can be traced in England and Wales. Already much decline had occurred; but since then this has been continuous. In the first decade the decrease amounted to 39 per cent contemporaneously with the introduction into towns of main sewerage schemes and still more of protected water-supplies. Then there was a lull in the rate of decline, followed by a decrease of nearly one-half between 1891–1900 and 1901–1910,

England and Wales. Average annual death-rate from enteric fever per million persons

1871–1880	1881–1890	1891–1900	1901–1910	1911–1920	1921–1925
332	198	174	91	35	25

and of not far from two-thirds between 1901–1910 and 1911–1920. If one may state categorically the influences working in these later decades, one would place first increasing protection of water-supplies and milk supplies from specific contamination; next to these the discovery that uncooked shell-fish, especially oysters and mussels were a common source of typhoid; and as powerful auxiliaries the detection of "carriers" of infection and the laboratory resources which have facilitated the diagnosis of the disease and the prompt taking of precautions.

But we must hark back to the earlier years when specific infectious diseases were regarded as developed within the community infected with them apart from any preceding case. In this connection we may quote a statement by Dr. Benjamin Rush (1745–1813) physician to the Pennsylvania Hospital, who was described by Lettsom, perhaps not extravagantly, as the American Sydenham.

Prior to the great epidemic of Yellow Fever in Philadelphia in the year 1793, Rush had taught that it only spread after importation; but in the light of experience of this terrible outbreak he faced contumely and hatred, and announced his conclusion that

> Philadelphia must admit the unwelcome truth sooner or later, that the Yellow Fever is engendered in her own bowels; or she must renounce her character for knowledge and policy, and perhaps with it her existence as a commercial city.

We now know that he was both right and wrong: for the Stegomyia fasciata which is the vector of Yellow Fever, must have bitten a Yellow Fever patient in or outside of Philadelphia, and have passed on the infection to human subjects in Philadelphia; furthermore if Philadelphia had not possessed around and in its houses stagnant water, suitable for breeding the stegomyia there would have been no general spread of the disease.

A further illustration of the doctrine as to the genesis of disease from dirt, reflecting the views of the English reformers, is contained in the following excerpt from the important report of the Massachusetts Sanitary Commission, 1850.

> Atmospheric contagion is generally harmless unless attracted by local causes . . . . that terrible disease, Asiatic Cholera, derives its terrific power chiefly or entirely from the accessory or accompanying circumstances which attend it. It bounds over habitation after habitation where cleanliness abides; . . . . while it alights near some congenial abode of filth or impurity. . . . . Wherever there is a dirty street, court, or dwelling-house, the elements of pestilence are at work in that neighbourhood.

And the important moral was drawn in the same report that

> The person who permits his neighbour's atmosphere to be contaminated by any filth . . . . is worse than a highway robber. The latter robs us of property, the former of life.

Similarly, Simon in England even earlier was teaching that

> In order to the prevention of Filth Diseases, the prevention of filth is indispensable;

And that there was need for local authorities

> To introduce for the first time, as into savage life, the rudiments of sanitary civilization.

This was sound teaching, except that it led to the persistence of the notion that offensive smells by themselves might be the cause of infectious disease. Against this notion John Snow made notable protest (see also page 145). Thus in a published letter, 1855, addressed to the President of the General Board of Health he refers to the attacks made upon him in medical and other journals on account of his evidence that certain offensive trades "do not cause, or in any way promote, the prevalence and mortality of cholera, fever, and other diseases, which are communicated from person to person." He goes on to quote the case of scabies, the prevalence of which, although greatest in the poor and dirty, is not ascribed to gases given off by decomposing matter, because its parasitic nature is known. While emphasising that he is "no defender of nuisances," he thinks that these should be dealt with by law, "without using the word pestiferous, or otherwise dragging in and distorting the science of medicine."

But although Snow took this enlightened and

advanced view, he nevertheless agreed with other hygienists that absence or defect of drainage "assists very much in the propagation of many epidemic diseases," and he pointed out the confusion of thought implied in confusing offensive smells from drainage with such smells from offensive trade processes. It need scarcely be stated that the latter smells may be obnoxious or injurious although incompetent to produce infectious disease.

At this point a crucial difference emerges. The school represented by Chadwick and Southwood Smith, and indeed the majority of sanitarians until recent decades, have attributed infectious diseases to effluvia from drains, closets, soil-pipes, etc., or even to accumulations of garbage. Snow in the letter quoted above with wonderful foresight protected himself against this view. He pointed out that drains removed all that comes from the sick, as well as from the healthy part of the community; and that when drains are defective, these matters might permeate the ground and pollute wells or other supplies of water. His view that specificity of contamination was needed to cause a typhoid infection is now generally accepted. It does not exclude possibilities in hot climates of infected matters being blown about in dust, or carried by flies; probably often carried in any climate on the feet or hands of children and others.

The persistence of the contrary view will be gathered from the quotations on pages 124 and 127. Those wishing to pursue the matter further cannot do better than consult the many illustrations given in the earlier pages of Murchison's masterly work on Continued Fevers. But there is one experience, that of Budd, which has secured the verdict against regarding typhoid fever as "pythogenic," the name given by Murchison, to indicate the putrefaction which he regarded as the souce of the fever.

Budd's investigations are embodied in his work on Typhoid Fever, 1873. Here we can give only the barest outline of his experiences and arguments, the teaching of which by him dated back as far as the year 1857. His argument is based on village experiences in which the course of events could be clearly traced. Summarily it is this: typhoid fever had been absent from a given village for years until introduced in 1855 by a young woman sent home ill from a neighbouring town. Then followed a number of cases in the girl's family, in neighbours who visited this family, or who used the same or neighbouring privies. The little community consisted of a few labourers' cottages clustered round two or three farmyards.

> In each of these were the usual manure yard and the inevitable pigsty; in each there was the same primitive accommodation for human needs. The same sun shown upon all alike, through month after month of the same dry, autumnal weather. From the soil of all, human and other exuviae exhaled into the air the same putrescent compounds. . . . . And yet, while at Loosebeare a large proportion of the inhabitants were lying prostrate with fever, in not one of the twenty or thirty exactly similar places was there a single case.

One differential fact explained matters; the arrival in the one hamlet of a girl sick with fever, from a town where at the time fever was rife.

Dr. Budd after describing his own experiences, quotes similar cases occurring in the year 1848, reported by Bretonneau and by de l'Eure in France, in which personal infection originated outbreaks of fever directly or indirectly through local fœcal contamination. He regarded sewers, as so-to-speak extensions of the human alimentary canal, spreading specific infection widely, and causing it to appear that the infection had its source in the sewer, and not in the already infected man. The link between the sewer and the patient infected from it was not clearly indicated; but, like Snow, it is possible that Budd was not thinking solely or even chiefly of water-contamination. He regarded putrid emanations from specifically infected material as able to infect through the air. We now know that sewage may infect not only water, but milk and such foods as oysters; and that an infected milkman may directly infect milk; but that in the absence of splashing, solid matters, including contagia, do not escape from liquids; and that until dust is produced or flies act as carriers, conveyance of infection from typhoid stools does not occur, apart from actual contact.

Milk has not infrequently been a vehicle for the infection of scarlet fever, diphtheria, and enteric fever. The first recorded instance is given in the *Edinburgh Medical Journal* for May, 1858, in a contribution by Dr. Michael W. Taylor, entitled "On the Communication of the Infection of Fever by Ingesta."

At this time typhus had not been generally distinguished from enteric fever, and Dr. Taylor writes of his cases as epidemic typhus, but as the first and infecting case only became convalescent at the end of the fourth week, this point causes no difficulty. E. O., a girl aged fifteen came home from Liverpool already ill with fever; two children in the same house fell ill a fortnight later with fever. The mother, who was the nurse, milked the cows, which supplied milk for fourteen families. In these families a series of cases of fever occurred; and from these other secondary cases originated. The particulars which cannot be detailed here are most convincing as to the infectivity of the milk. The same observer in 1867 shewed that scarlet fever might be spread in the same way, and in more recent years many outbreaks of these two diseases, of diphtheria, and of septic sore throat have been traced to milk supplies. In some of these outbreaks a human source of infection has failed to be traced, and suspicion not completely sustained, except perhaps for diphtheria, has been aroused that the cow may suffer from illness causing the same disease in man. The chief disease which has been proved to be spread by milk from a diseased cow is tuberculosis of bovine origin, tuberculosis of the glands or bones or mesenteric disease being sometimes caused in this way.

CHAPTER XVII

The Prevention of Cholera

Although cholera is an exotic disease outside its home and starting place in India, it has repeatedly invaded Western countries with devastating results. Neither as regards this disease, nor it may be added Plague, have we complete knowledge of the reasons determining its peregrinations westward, with an activity which (as in Plague) appears to indicate increased carrying power arising from factors at present hidden from us. But, whatever may be these factors of pandemicity, we know that both Plague and Cholera can be completely controlled, and pandemicity as well as endemicity of these diseases may be made to disappear from the face of the earth by measures well within our powers.

Cholera as an exotic disease would naturally be left out of the limited view attempted in this volume, were it not for the consideration that it is in connection with cholera and "fever"—the two were viewed from the same angle by the earlier sanitary reformers—that our chief sanitary triumphs have been achieved; and it is in connection with the same diseases that the contest as to specific or non-specific causation of infectious diseases has been largely fought out.

In this matter four names stand out, as having had—at least so far as Britain and America are concerned—the maximum influence in determining the course of events which has led to or impeded the elimination of cholera and typhoid fever from temperate countries, viz., John Snow, William Budd, Max von Pettenkofer, and John Simon. The two first named of these must be counted to be the greatest of English epidemiologists; and their contribution to the elucidation of the law that specific infection is the sole source of cholera and typhoid fever, so far as can be judged by English experience, has been of fundamental importance in the history of preventive medicine.

John Snow (1813–1858) practised medicine in London, his chief work for many years being that of an anaesthetist. By his scientific investigations and his development of satisfactory methods, he ranks as a chief founder of the science and practice of anaesthesia. Some of the following facts are taken from B. W. Richardson's prefatory memoir to Snow's work *On Chloroform and Other Anaesthetics*, 1857, and from the account of Snow contained in the *Asclepiad*, 1887, also by Richardson. In 1831–1832 Snow had seen many cases of cholera in Newcastle-on-Tyne, and in 1848 again turned his thoughts to the same subject. He inferred from its clinical features that the poison of cholera is taken directly into the alimentary canal by the mouth; and began to suspect water as the chief, though not the only, medium for conveying this poison, which he concluded was derived from the excreted matter of the cholera patient. In 1849 he published his views in a pamphlet entitled "The Mode of Communication of Cholera." This "peculiar doctrine" as Simon described it (p. 443 in Vol. I of Simon's reprinted *Public Health Reports*, 1887), was but the preliminary to systematic investigation in the great epidemic of cholera in London in 1854. I have not space here to give details of the well-known outbreak of cholera chiefly occurring among the consumers of water from the Broad Street pump. The best account of this outbreak, apart from the original report, is given in Chapter VIII of Sedgwick's *Principles of Sanitary Science and the Public Health*, 1902. Snow was not content with this demonstration—as nearly conclusive as an investigation could be in the absence of our present machinery of notification of cases, trained house-to-house investigators, and so on. For a time in Richardson's words: "he laid aside as much as possible the emoluments of practice, and when (he could not do all the work himself) he paid for qualified labour." He thus ascertained in 1854 the distribution of deaths from cholera in the south districts of the metropolis. In the area supplied with drinking water from one Company's sources 288, in the area of a second Company 71, and in a third area 5 deaths from cholera occurred to each 10,000 houses, this corresponding with the part of the River Thames from which each Company derived its water, according to the degree of pollution of its waters. Richardson claims for Snow, and I think correctly, "the entire originality of the communication of cholera by the direct introduction of the excreted cholera poison into the alimentary system; but independently of that theory, the entire originality of the discovery of a connection between impure water supply and choleraic disease." It is noteworthy that a 2nd edition of his work on the *Mode of Communication of Cholera*, 1855, in which Snow summarised the whole of his observations, is recorded by Richardson as costing him £200 in preparation and publication, and realizing in return scarcely so many shillings.

We may add here a reference to Snow's presidential oration to the Medical Society of London in 1853, which confirms Snow's supremely high position as an epidemiologist. The subject taken was "Continuous Molecular Changes, more particularly in their relation to Epidemic Diseases." In this address Dr. Snow used the word "communicable" "in preference to contagious for various reasons." He drew attention to the fact that "the material cause of every communicable disease resembles a species of living being in this, that both one and the other depend on, and in fact consist of, a series of continuous molecular changes, occurring in suitable materials."

Speaking on the communicability of diseases Dr. Snow said that "the communication of diseases was not generally recognized until a recent period. Even

Sydenham did not recognize the communicability of any acute febrile disease except the plague. He did not even recognize the communicability of small-pox. Sydenham, however, was fully aware of the resemblance between the material causes of an epidemic disease and the species of animal or plant, but he was not aware that animals and plants proceed only from procreation by their own kind."

Reference was made in the same address to Professor Schonbein's discovery of ozone. It was straightway supposed that this was the cause of cholera. Later when ozone was found to be pretty generally present, cholera and some other diseases were attributed to its absence!

When the communication of diseases began to be recognized, it was thought to depend, in most cases, on effluvia given off from the patient into the surrounding air; even syphilis, for some time after its appearance in Europe, was believed to be propagated in this way, and persons suffering from it were driven out of the towns and villages to live or die in the fields, lest they should infect others with their breath, although the disease was not attributed to any misconduct on their part.

Dr. Snow's views on predisposition of any disease are worthy of quotation.

Until it can be shewn that the materies morbi of any communicable disease has really entered the economy of those who do not take the malady, there is no reason to invoke a supposed predisposition, or predisposing causes, to account for its existence in the persons in whom we find it. To be of the human species, and to receive the morbid poison in a suitable manner, is most likely all that is required.

William Budd (1811–1880) as already noted (p. 161) in 1849 had already advanced views as to the specificity of the cholera infection which were identical with those of Snow. In a later publication (*Memoranda on Asiatic Cholera, its Mode of Spreading, and its Prevention*, 1865) he made the following statement:

The evidence adduced in these documents, is intended to support the theory that Asiatic Cholera is propagated exclusively by the characteristic discharges from the intestinal canal of persons affected with it; and further to show, that, under given conditions, the spread of the disease may be prevented by a plan which I was *the first to suggest and employ*, so long ago as *1849:*—viz., by *destroying by disinfectants*, the specific powers of these discharges, immediately on their issue from the body.

In a final paragraph he made the following statements:

I cannot conclude this memorandum without drawing attention to the very important works on the same subject by the late Dr. Snow.

I was led to the principal opinions I hold, respecting the propagation of Cholera, before the appearance of his first Memoir, and on entirely independent grounds. I had also taught, for many years, at the Bristol Medical School, the leading doctrines regarding the propagation of Typhoid Fever, which are enumerated in the series of papers herewith enclosed. But Dr. Snow was the first to announce publicly that Asiatic Cholera is disseminated by the rice-water discharges, and to substantiate the statement by evidence which, for my own part, I consider to be perfectly conclusive.

It will be seen, then, that both Snow and Budd arrived independently at the same conclusion, a conclusion which is now everywhere accepted.

Although it belongs rather to Chapter XVIII, allusion may be made here to the practice of "Disinfection by Anticipation" for both domestic and municipal purposes, urged by Budd, who said that "when epidemics were threatened, no house should be without these precious safeguards;" and he claimed that in the experience of Bristol in the Cholera invasion of 1866 the outbreak had been curtailed by disinfection of the excreta of the sick, of latrines and of sewers. Budd's investigations on enteric fever are summarised in Chapter XVII.

Before discussing the important official reports of John Simon, it is convenient here to indicate the place of Pettenkofer in the development of preventive medicine, especially as bearing on the spread of cholera and enteric fever.

Max von Pettenkofer (1818–1901) during the earlier part of his professional life was working on the problems of physiological chemistry and metabolism. He investigated problems of ventilation of dwelling-houses, of clothing, and of the soil, and may be rightly described as the founder of experimental hygiene. From 1855 onwards, as Professor of Hygiene at Munich, he made continuous studies of the etiology of cholera and typhoid fever, with which we are chiefly concerned here. After a study of the invasion of Bavaria by Cholera in 1854, and the distribution of the disease, he abandoned the view of direct infection generally accepted, and his views were widely regarded as authoritative. The full statement of his theory was published in *Zum Gegenwartigen Stand der Cholerafrage* in 1887. At the age of 74 he swallowed a culture of virulent cholera bacilli in support of his theory that some change of the contagium of the disease in the soil was necessary in the initiation of the disease. The evidence collected by him appeared to show that the spread of cholera did not follow the lines of human intercourse, but was confined to the vicinity of streams and rivers. These localities were found to present certain conditions of soil—porosity, moisture and organic pollution—which he regarded as essential for a widespread development of the virus of cholera. He failed to find any connection between water supply and cholera in Munich, although the distribution of the many water supplies in the city made inquiry in this direction easy. According to Pettenkofer, a district is most prone to choleraic infection when the groundwater is sinking in porous soil, this constituting his "zeitliche Predisposition." He did not exclude the importation of infection by a cholera patient as forming part of the causation of an epidemic of cholera. Thus in his report to the Cholera Commission of the German Empire (English Translation,

1876) he describes himself as "holding fast to the principle that the distribution of cholera from place to place is effected by human intercourse;" and referring to the frequent instances in which such importation could not be discovered, he gives the warning statement that "the fact can only warrant the assumption, that the infected persons and the intercourse with them are not the sole causes at work." His view was that a part of the life-history of the contagium must take place in the soil, this needing certain conditions of the soil to make it potent. He thus appeared to exclude direct infection from patient to patient as causing cholera. In his own words cholera was neither wholly a contagion nor wholly a miasm, but a bastard of the two. It is probable that had these views not received general acceptance, and still more had not the earlier sanitary leaders, Chadwick and Southwood Smith, been so "anti-contagionist" in their views, more rapid progress might have been realized. Pettenkofer's views had great influence on the policy of sanitary advisers in England, and must, I think, be credited with responsibility for the inadequate emphasis which in the earlier years was placed on the special sanitary improvement, viz., a perfectly safe water supply, which would bring about the most rapid reduction of disease. On the other hand, it is arguable that the general campaign against filth urged with unrivalled eloquence and force by Simon, and forming the main item in the sanitary work of Chadwick and Southwood Smith, was remarkably effective also in securing clean supplies of water for the public. For a balanced judgment on this point, Simon's official reports to the Privy Council must be consulted. My opinion is stated above. A few illustrations may be given here.

In 1853 a Committee appointed by the President of the General Board of Health and consisting of Drs. Arnott, Baly, Farr, Owen and Simon, while feeling "bound to express themselves with some reserve," because of the absence of circumstantial proof of the connection of infected water with cholera; added "the present state of knowledge does not justify dogmatic assertions on this subject; but . . . . the slightest taint of organic contamination within the drinking water of a large population constitutes a danger which we cannot but regard with as much alarm as disgust." There was a gradual advance from the anti-contagionism of Southwood Smith's position; and Simon in his official reports reiterated his main teaching that "in the districts which suffer the high diarrhœal death-rates, the population either breathes or drinks a large amount of putrefying animal refuse" (1858). In a footnote to the report of 1858 is a statement by Simon, added apparently by him at the time of the issue of his reprinted reports in 1887. In this note Simon, after summarizing in an appreciative manner Snow's teaching in 1849–1855, as to the direct propagation of cholera, adds that "whatever may be the worth of the theory, it has been of use in contributing to draw attention to the vast hygienic importance of a pure water-supply."

Simon then in the same reprint draws attention to experiments made in 1854 by Professor Thiersch of Erlangen on mice, which appeared to shew that cholera evacuations acquire contagiousness in the course of their decomposition. Budd, in his work on *Typhoid Fever*, 1873, p. 91, also quotes these experiments, which were used to shew that "the poison of typhoid fever is not cast off from the body in a finished state;" and remarks that they would be decisive if it were proved that the mice poisoned by putrefied choleraic excretions had the power to communicate cholera to other mice. This was wanting. Murchison some years later taught the necessity for a maturation of infection for typhoid evacuations. Simon drew a hopeful lesson from these experiments and from observations by Acland at Oxford and by Pettenkofer at Munich that an outbreak of cholera followed the immigration of a choleraic patient. Simon contrasted smallpox in which direct infection occurs, and cholera in which "if truly the disease be contagious, foulness of medium seems indispensable." The lesson here drawn was sound, except that the direct infectivity of cholera appears to be doubted or excluded; for given completely satisfactory excretal arrangements and a pure water supply (with protection of milk and such foods as oysters from exposure to excretal matter) the possibility of a considerable outbreak of cholera—as also of typhoid fever—is eliminated. But the serious defect in the teaching of Pettenkofer was that direct infection of attendant or nurse by the patient was excluded; and by similar reasoning the influence of chronic or intermittent "carriers" in infecting healthy persons, subsequently ascertained, would also have been excluded.

Writing in his official report for 1866 Simon again expressed his conviction that cholera derives all its epidemic destructiveness from filth, and especially from excremental uncleanliness, a perfectly sound statement; but rendered less quickly efficient in preventive medicine than it would otherwise have been, had Simon accepted fully Snow's teaching, and directed preponderant attention to the urgent need for pure water supplies. This he did, but as indicated above, his statements were handicapped. He could not do this because of his acceptance, in common with the majority of his contemporaries, of Pettenkofer's theories, which subsequent events have shewn to be unfounded. Those wishing to pursue this subject further will find the necessary references in Vol. II of the Sanitary Institute's Reprint of Simon's reports. We may, in conclusion, quote from a note by Simon (1866) on page 319 of this reprint:

> I must repeat my deep sense of the value of Prof. v. Pettenkofer's researches. . . . . It appears certain that hence-

forth no local health officer will be properly up to the standard of his scientific duties, unless he thoroughly knows the distribution and stratification of soils in the district for which he acts, nor unless he also maintains such systematic and exact observation of the heights of wells as will enable him always to speak with precision as to the movements of water-level in the soil; for it seems established that these are two great governing influences in relation to the spread of disease.

Such knowledge is valuable from other points of view; but the general abandonment of Pettenkofer's teaching reduces the above statement, in relation to preventive medicine, to a lower level of value.

In 1866 (see *Report to Privy Council*, pp. 366 and 457) Simon regarded the distribution of cholera in London as appearing to illustrate and to be explained by Pettenkofer's ground-water theory. In this connection may be mentioned Farr's report on the epidemic of cholera in 1849, in which it was shewn that the death-rate from this disease in different parts of London was greatest in the parts nearest the river and decreased progressively as the altitude increased. This was explained by Farr not on Pettenkofer's hypothesis, but was believed by Farr to depend on gravitation of choleraic material. These gropings after truth were a necessary stage in the advance of the science of preventive medicine.

CHAPTER XVIII

Disinfection in Preventive Medicine

In tracing the course of preventive medicine, it is important to remember that at every stage human necessity activated by fear and panic was urging the adoption of preventive measures. Imperfect and incomplete knowledge was no justification for inaction in the face of a great calamity; and the public which demanded active measures had no conception of the flimsy basis of knowledge on which the advice of ancient and mediaeval physicians was necessarily based.

The necessary dependence of preventive on clinical medicine cannot be more clearly illustrated than in the preventive measures adopted up to comparatively recent years. These measures were almost indiscriminately applied to any epidemic disease; as was inevitable, until the natural history of each specific infectious disease, including a knowledge of special channels and vectors of infection in each disease, was discovered by observation and experiment. The following instances relating to chemical purification will illustrate some of the stages in progress and a little of the waste of effort before exact knowledge of each disease was available.

There is a close connection between ancient knowledge of antiseptics and chemical agents aimed at preventing disease. Both Hebrews and Greeks employed antiseptics in their religious rites. Dr. J. Campbell Brown (*History of Chemistry*, 1913) illustrates the high degree of skill in the use of antiseptics attained in Egypt by the fact that the body of King Rameses (B.C. 1300) was preserved so completely as to enable his features to be photographed as clearly as if they had been buried not more than a week.

Rhazes, the greatest of Arabian physicians (A.D. 860–932), (Dr. E. G. Browne, Arabian Medicine, *Fitzpatrick Lectures*, 1921), when asked for the most suitable site for a hospital, is stated to have caused pieces of meat to be hung up in different parts of the town and chosen the place where decomposition was the slowest.

The action of Hippocrates in attempting to fumigate Athens has already been noted (p. 57), and more modern attempts at Marseilles are quoted on page 78.

So long as pestilence was attributed to a general putrid condition of the air, actuated by occult terrestrial or astral influences, attempts at disinfection must necessarily have been little more than experiments of despair; but when it began to be suspected that for the occurrence of fermentation and putrefaction the presence in the air of organized forms of life was necessary, disinfection became more nearly practical. An early expression of this view is contained in the writings of Bishop Berkeley (1685–1753) the apostle of immaterialism. In 1744 he published a treatise on the virtues of tar water, which in his opinion was a cure for the blood impurities in pleurisy, pneumonia, erysipelas and other diseases, and even a preventive of smallpox. His views were satirised by O. W. Holmes, who said, Berkeley "held two very odd opinions; that tar water was everything and that the whole material word was nothing." The Bishop died suddenly, and as Holmes said, a little unkindly: "there was not time enough to stir up a quart of his panacea."

Even before Berkeley's time disinfection in the form of fumigation of rooms had become a trade. Shakespeare makes one of his characters say, "I was entertained for a perfumer when I was smoking a fusty room;" and vinegar and various aromatics were used as preventives of infection. Doctors carried aromatics in their gold-headed cane; and a sprig of rue was placed on the bench near the Judge in the hope of warding off infection. Destruction of bedding and apparel and even of dwellings was practised in some pestilences. The futility of most of the measures of domiciliary disinfection formerly practised may be illustrated by the extract below from the report of the Council of Hygiene of New York, setting out the failure to act effectively during the epidemic of Smallpox in 1865 (quoted from Mapother's *Lectures on Public Health*, 1867, p. 509).

It is stated that in only two instances out of 1,200 cases of this disease were visits made by inspectors of the city government. In one instance

> The so-called health warden stopped at the foot of a stairway forty feet distant from the poor tenant who had the disease, and delivered his orders as follows: "Put pieces of camphor about the clothing of those who are not sick, and occasionally throw some camphor upon the hot stove."

Reference has been made to the importance attaching to the discovery that "fever" included two distinct diseases. There followed on this a gradual discovery of the different methods of spread of these diseases; typhus by "emanations" from the sick, and typhoid by swallowing infected material discharged from the alimentary canal. There was an earlier stage in which it was believed that effluvia from intestinal discharges could spread infection (p. 137); though it was thought not until fermentative changes had occurred in these; and as regards typhus it has more recently been discovered that typhus spreads, and probably spreads solely when lice from a typhus patient infest a healthy person who has been in contact with this patient or his apparel.

The discovery of these facts has rendered the prevention of typhoid and typhus possible on accurate lines, for which complete success can be promised. Thus

Prevention of typhoid fever:

1. Disinfect all discharges from patient
2. Perfect cleanliness of attendants on the sick
3. Dispose of these discharges in such a manner that they cannot obtain access to any water or food supplies
4. Use modern methods of prompt diagnosis of doubtful cases of typhoid
5. Search for "carrier" cases

Prevention of typhus fever:

1. Isolation of the patient under a skilled nurse
2. Disinfestation of patient and of his personal and bed linen, etc.
3. Disinfestation and surveillance of "contacts" for 14 to 21 days
4. General attack on pediculosis. The practice of cleanliness

The above scheme is set out to indicate the chief lines of action on which typhoid and typhus can now be reduced to insignificance. The relation of the indicated lines of action to past efforts will be seen as we proceed.

Reference may be made to the chemical safeguard against infection by water which have been introduced in the last few years (p. 41).

In the past, even since the sanitary renaissance, vast sums of money have been spent on "futile libations and powderings" in attempting to control our common infectious diseases. Gaseous fumigations still maintain their utility in certain cases, as by sulphurous acid or hydrocyanic acid (with very special precautions) in freeing the holds of ships from rats. Chemical purification of rooms in smallpox is also valuable; and disinfection by heat in the form of steam has become an established practice in disinfecting contaminated bedding, clothing and woollen goods, as in smallpox and anthrax, or in disinfestation of these from lice. That a great heat, like that of an oven, effectually destroys infection in all substances exposed to it for some time was stated by Lind in his *Observations on the Jail Distemper*, 1779. The heat of an oven, he said, had "a destroying power which no infection whatever can resist." He also made the point that, when once contagion is present, no ventilation or admission of air into prisons or hospitals can remove or destroy it; an essentially important fact of which most writers in the early sanitary period were ignorant.

The story of the award by Parliament of a large money grant to Dr. Carmichael Smyth in 1795 for his discovery of the value of nitrous acid fumes in destroying infection may be recalled. Particulars are given in his volume *The Effect of the Nitrous Vapour in preventing and destroying Contagion*, 1799. There can be little doubt that the nitrous fumes, used as they were in crowded hospital ships, were useful in diminishing infection, though the measure in the light of our present knowledge must be regarded as only incidentally successful. Cleanliness of patients, freeing them from infestation by vermin, and segregation of the sick we now know would have rendered superfluous the use of a feeble agent such as domestic fumigation. Smyth's volume is interesting as shewing the then view of communicable diseases. Two classes were described, viz. *specific contagions* like smallpox and measles, which "do not arise from any general quality or process of nature with which we are acquainted;" and *general contagions*, which may be named "putrid," as they result from one of those general "fermentative processes to which water as well as all vegetable and animal substances, under certain circumstances, are liable." Smyth adds that the conclusion that jail or hospital fever derives its origin from the latter source "admits of every species of evidence which a matter of fact and observation can do."

Two further illustrations of disinfection may be taken from the writings of Dr. William Budd (1811–1880) of Bristol. In a pamphlet on "Scarlet Fever," of which the fifth edition, 1881, is here quoted, Dr. Budd proposed the rational means for preventing the spread of this fever, which is "to annihilate the germs proceeding from these various sources" (throat and nose "especially virulent," kidney, bowels and skin), "on their very issue from the body, and before the patient leaves the sick-room." This was a scientific proposition; and both in this disease and in diphtheria, measles and all catarrhal affections, the recommendation is sound. Dr. Budd thought that discharges from scarlatinal patients into sewers were the source of serious infection, presumably by aerial effluvia from these sewers. This we now know is not so; neither typhoid fever, cholera nor scarlet fever being communicable by effluvia (which are entirely gaseous, apart from splashing) from excretal discharges, but only by these discharges when hands are dirtied, or the discharges gain entrance into drinking water, milk or other food. Here a point of distinction arises; for scarlet fever has never, and cholera and typhoid fever have frequently been traced to contaminated drinking water. The need for exact knowledge of the life-history of each disease is evident, and this has only been secured by slow and painful stages. Similarly owing to its large surface, Budd thought that "the crop of new poison which escapes by the skin probably far exceeds in amount that which escapes by the other surfaces." In smallpox almost certainly this is the case; in scarlet fever the balance of evidence is against this view, and favours the conclusion that protracted infection and recurrence of infection in scarlet fever are associated with the lurking and continued multiplication of the contagium in the naso-pharyngeal passages.

An earlier paper on "Malignant Cholera," written by Dr. Budd in 1849 illustrates another aspect of the same subject. After stating his conclusion that "the human intestine is the sole breeding-place of the poison" of this disease, he pointed out the "momentous practical consequences to which" (this conclusion) "directly leads." For instance, if on the first invasion of this disease into England, "the poison contained in the discharges of infected persons had been destroyed (and the destruction of it may doubtless be accomplished by simple means), *malignant cholera had never been epidemic in England;*" and he added that even after its admission, "we may yet abridge its sojourn among us." He recommended chloride of zinc solution (Burnett's fluid) for the double task of immediate disinfection of all infected discharges, and for disinfection of the contents of sewers, and offensive matter elsewhere. Even at this early stage Budd recognized that "water is the principal medium through which cholera diffuses itself," but he added "we must look to the air to explain its occasional transport" over wide tracts, its introduction into new countries, and often to explain single and casual cases.

Scabies is interesting as the simplest illustration of the operation of disinfection, i.e., of destruction of a specific cause of disease by physical or chemical means. In the case of action against pediculi and acari it is called disinfestation. Scabies was formerly regarded as evidence of constitutional dyscrasia; and Sydenham in prescribing for it, ordered first a bolus containing roots of Virginian snakeweed and

Oriental Bezoar-stone to be taken for one to twenty days, followed each morning by waters of Carduus Benedictus. "If the pustules do not yet vanish," a sulphur ointment was to be applied to the affected parts. We now know that this application without the preceding internal treatment would effect a rapid cure. Garrison states that Avenzoar, who died in 1162, described the itch-mite. Bonomo also described this parasite in 1687. That this knowledge was slow in acceptance is illustrated by the following extract from Dr. Thomas Marryat's *Therapeutics or the Art of Healing*, (20th edition, 1805), in which he describes the cause of the Itch as being "an infectious miasma sui generis;" adding "the hypothesis of its being wholly owing to animalcules is highly doubtful." Pringle in his *Observations on the Diseases of the Army*, (6th ed. 1768), gives (p. 346) a footnote crediting Bonomo as being the first who proposed curing the itch by external applications only." Pringle mentions the practical point (in the absence of arrangements for disinfection of clothing by heat) that the method of cure by sulphur inunction "oftener fails with the officers than with the men; because the latter having no change of dress, what they wore was purified by the medicine, at the same time that they themselves were cured; whilst the former, catching the itch, have sometimes kept it longer, from the circulation of infection between their body and their clothes."

The Great War (1914–1918) brought out the momentous importance of disinfestation as a means of preventing disease and increasing military efficiency. As this disinfestation is secured by chemical and physical means, brief reference may be made here to the experience of the Great War.

Body lice have been known for some years to be the vectors of typhus fever and relapsing fever; and it was discovered during the Great War that Trench Fever—one of the largest single causes of disability of soldiers—is also conveyed by lice. In 1917 in the Second Army of the British Forces one-fifth of the total admissions to the casualty clearing stations were found to be the result of Trench Fever. Hence bathing and disinfestation of clothing and bedding, on a rigid and universal scale for all suspects, by means of dry or moist heat would, had it been practicable, have greatly reduced the drain on man-power. Similar remarks apply to the early detection and the treatment of scabies by the application of sulphur ointment or of liquor calcis sulphuratae. The terrible losses of Napoleon's Army on its retreat from Moscow were due largely to typhus fever; and the Great War on its eastern side provided even more portentous evidence of the importance of disinfestation. Thus in *Typhus Fever with particular Reference to the Serbian Epidemic*, 1920, by Dr. R. P. Strong, and collaborators, it is stated that in the epidemic of typhus which occurred in 1915 over 150,000 deaths occurred within six months before the epidemic could be suppressed.

The lesson from the preceding illustrations is that disinfection if it is to be "worth while" must be specifically directed to a definite end, this end being based on accurate knowledge of the natural history, including the method of spread, of the disease which is being dealt with.

CHAPTER XIX

Immunisation against Infection

A. SMALL-POX INOCULATION

In our survey of the past, so far as it has been accomplished in preceding chapters, we have been concerned chiefly with the advances of knowledge which have rendered it possible to control certain infectious diseases. There came first the very slow realization of the fact that these diseases were communicable from person to person, a realization which until recent years was tempered and belittled by persistent belief that infection only occurred when there was a pestilential condition of the air (not of human origin) and possibly also when the body humours were in a disordered condition. For a large number of these diseases we now know that no such necessary association exists. We know now that typhus can be entirely abolished, given personal cleanliness in the entire community. We know that enteric fever and cholera cannot obtain a footing in any community if supplies of water and food are protected. We know that, given drainage of marshes and the avoidance of stagnant pools, and if with this we also prevent the attack of mosquitos on patients suffering from malaria or yellow fever, these diseases can be annihilated. There are other diseases against which our efforts are relatively ineffective, particularly those which are conveyed largely if not chiefly or solely by infectious material discharged from the naso-pharynx and the lungs, e.g., measles, whooping cough, poliomyelitis, encephalitis lethargica, meningococcal fever, pneumonia. There are many tropical and subtropical diseases aginst which recent knowledge opens out the prospect of complete control through exact biological knowledge. What has already been done in the control of hookworm disease, a disease which in some countries is more devastating in its results than even malaria or tuberculosis or syphilis, is well known. By the practice of elementary sanitation, scientifically applied, along with treatment of individual patients, this disease can be entirely controlled. The methods of control of tuberculosis and syphilis must be left for later consideration.

But so far as concerns the more common infectious diseases prevailing in western Europe and in America, the chief means for prevention which have hitherto emerged have been

1. The sanitation of domestic dwellings, including prompt removal of waste matters from the house, and the provision of drainage and sewerage for villages and towns,

2. The purification and protection of water supplies and of foods from recurrent contamination by organic filth;

3. The diminution of domestic overcrowding;

4. The institutional segregation of the infectious sick;

5. The disinfection and cleansing of infected rooms, bedding, clothing, etc.

These measures, as we have seen, until recent years were regarded as almost equally applicable to all infectious diseases; and the differentiation of these diseases and enlightenment as to their individual methods of spread meant an important advance in the possibilities of prevention.

Among the diseases against which protection was most urgently needed was Small Pox. This disease has been one of the greatest scourges of mankind for many ages. The first clear account of it is contained in Rhazes' treatise on the Small Pox, written about A.D. 900, when already Small Pox was a well-known disease.

Like Influenza and some other diseases (page 72) Small Pox at irregular intervals shews an unwonted ability to spread and become pandemic, as in the European outbreaks of 1838 and of 1870–1873. For particulars as to the epidemiology of Small Pox my contribution in the *British Medical Journal*, July 5, 1902 may be consulted, in which I remark:

> As the expression of a fact, without being committed to a theory we may admit with the older epidemiologists that there is a *constitutio epidemica variolosa*. What is meant by this is that at certain irregular intervals Small Pox, as judged by its wider spread, is more infectious than it is in other years

with equal opportunities for its dissemination. There is no regular periodicity for these greater epidemics.

The extent of prevalence and the mortality from Small Pox are illustrated by many facts to be gathered from medical writings and parish registers of deaths in the eighteenth century.

Thus Dr. Robert Watt (*An Inquiry into the Relative Mortality of the Principal Diseases of Children in Glasgow*, 1813) found on investigating the Parish registers of Glasgow during the preceding thirty years that more than half of the total deaths occurred under ten years of age, and that "of this half more than one-third" (i.e., one-sixth of the total deaths) "died of the Small Pox." Dividing the thirty years into five equal periods the percentage proportion of deaths from Small Pox to total deaths in successive periods 1783–1788 to 1807–1812, was 19.6, 18.2, 18.7, 8.9, 3.9.

From the same source is obtained the following abstract of the experience of London derived from its Bills of Mortality:

	1700–1711	1710–1721	1720–1731	1730–1741	1740–1751	1750–1761	1760–1771	1770–1781	1780–1791	1790–1801
Proportion per cent of deaths from small pox to total deaths.......	5.7	8.0	8.4	7.7	7.2	10.3	10.3	9.6	9.2	9.4

Dr. John Haygarth (in *A Sketch of a Plan to Exterminate the Casual Small Pox from Great Britain and to introduce General Inoculation*, 1793) gives a number of statistics as to small pox. He quotes French estimates to the effect that one in ten of all children born died of small pox, and cites Baron Dimsdale, Dr. Percival, and other authorities as stating that in London birth are to deaths from small pox in the proportion of $6\frac{1}{4}$ to one, in Manchester $6\frac{1}{2}$ to one, in Liverpool $5\frac{1}{2}$ to one, and in Chester $6\frac{2}{3}$ to one.

In the east it had long been known that inoculation of small pox virus under favourable conditions produced a milder attack than disease arising from infection naturally derived. In 1718 Lady Mary Wortley Montagu had her son inoculated successfully in Adrianople; in 1722, two members of the British royal family were similarly inoculated, and the practice rapidly spread. In 1768 Dr. Dimsdale inoculated Catherine, Empress of Russia; and between 1750 and the introduction of vaccination by William Jenner in 1799, a large part of the total population was inoculated. By improved procedures the risk of death from the inoculated disease was very greatly reduced; but in the absence of strict isolation of the inoculated, they became a source of danger to all who were not similarly inoculated, or who had not suffered from natural small pox. That this danger was realised, is evidenced in Dr. Thomas Bateman's *Reports on the Diseases of London, 1804 to 1816.*

Thus on page 92, Bateman says: "They who circulate the poison seem to forget or to disregard the mischief of partial inoculation, and the numbers which they weekly contribute to swell the bills of mortality." On page 98 he speaks of decreasing small pox in one year, and adds that it would probably have disappeared during the cold season, "had not the poison been extensively circulated by inoculation." On page 200 he mentions those (referring to Mr. Brick's *Serious Reasons for uniformly opposing Vaccination*, 1807) who complacently urge that the small pox is "a merciful provision of Providence for the poor man, by diminishing the burden of his family."

Inoculated small pox undoubtedly was much less severe than the natural disease; but with the discovery of vaccination it became unjustifiable and in 1840 was made illegal. Even before this, and long before any special public health law regarding infection was enacted, objection was taken to inoculation under the common law of the land, as an infringement of the fundamental principle *sic utere tuo, ut alienum non laedas;* and a doctor and a patient were both fined for not taking the necessary steps to prevent an inoculated patient coming into contact with others. Dr. Bateman's remarks on this point—in view of later public health activities—may cause a smile.

The general interference of government in our domiciliary concerns is doubtless to be deprecated; but, while we submit our sea-faring men to the outlawry of the quarantine (for its severity almost warrants that title), we can see no possible objection, on the grounds of despotic interference, to compelling those who *will* receive the variolous contagion, to confine its sphere to their own houses and to restraining public institutions.

Prior to Jenner's discovery this was the position. Small pox was so prevalent that few escaped disfigurement and many died. By inoculation in favourable circumstances a mild attack could be obtained. By segregating the inoculated it was possible to prevent them from becoming a public danger. It is not surprising therefore that general, as distinguished from sporadic, inoculation was advocated. As Dr. William Heberden put it in his *Observations on the Increase and Decrease of Certain Diseases*, 1801:

> While the inoculation of the wealthy keeps up a perpetual source of infection, many others, who either cannot afford, or do not chuse, to adopt the same method, are continually exposed to the distemper. . . . . There must always be an objection against making any great city the place for inoculation, until the practice is become universal among all ranks of people.

A bold effort was made to secure the universal adoption of inoculation at Chester in England. It owed its genesis to Dr. Haygarth, who set out the arguments for his proposal, in certain propositions which may be summarised in the statements that small pox is infectious; it has never been known, since its original commencement, to be produced by any other cause than infection; it is communicable through the medium of the air; it can only be conveyed in the near vicinity of the patient, or by means of contaminated clothes, etc. After discussing these points, Haygarth quotes a letter from Dr. Benjamin Waterhouse, who had lived for some years in Rhode Island in America. The particulars given in this letter are valuable evidence of the early adoption of severe measures of quarantine and isolation for small pox patients. Inoculation had been discouraged both in Boston and Rhode Island; and as contrasted with the experience of London, in which during the 17th and 18th centuries small pox was constantly endemic, and frequently epidemic, may be given that of Boston, in which epidemics of small pox occurred,

In 1666, after an absence of 17 years
In 1678, after an absence of 12 years
In 1689, after an absence of 11 years
In 1702, after an absence of 13 years
In 1721, after an absence of 19 years
In 1730, after an absence of 9 years
In 1752, after an absence of 22 years

In such circumstances of infrequent importation of the disease, quarantine and segregation were the best policy, and inoculation in some parts of America was wisely avoided.

Haygarth's Chester plan had been referred to Dr. John Fothergill in 1778, who shewed it to his friends. These, he says, gave it a mixed reception "in proportion to their humanity." The scheme consisted in short in the proposal to provide inoculation for all, and to arrange for domestic instead of hospital segregation, thus avoiding undue expense. Public inoculators were to be appointed, paid out of public subscriptions, 5/– being suggested as the inoculator's fee, and 2/– being given to indigent parents for nursing each inoculated child. It was proposed that a general inoculation should be made at intervals of two years or longer, arranged so as to prevent the occurrence of natural small pox in children. It was also arranged that a monetary reward should be given within a month after the disappearance of infection to the parents of the infected family, when after periodical inspection, it was certified that they had used all the prescribed methods for preventing the infection of neighbours, etc. Furthermore, reward was given to those reporting unknown cases of small pox. Haygarth after summarising the favourable local results of his scheme, draws the inference that "there might safely and successfully be founded a general law to promote inoculation, or, what would be incomparably more easy, and more grateful to the feelings of humanity, to establish regulations that would *exterminate the small pox from Great Britain.*"

In the preceding greatly abbreviated sketch, we have seen what were the first serious attempts made to control small pox. They consisted in isolation of patients, either at home or in Houses of Recovery, in the enforcement of measures of quarantine (in American ports), in the fumigation and cleansing of

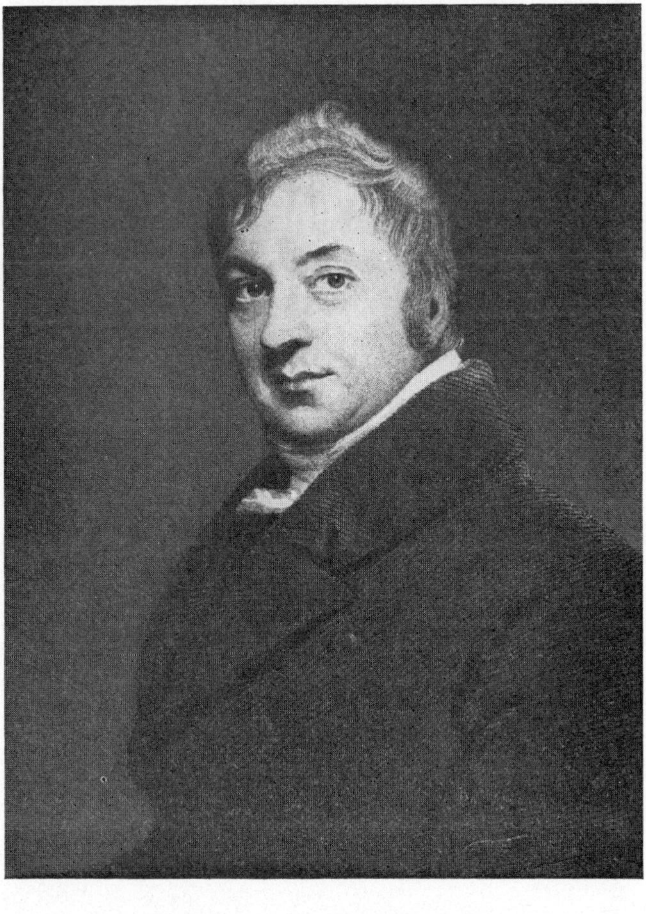

Edward Jenner (1749–1823)

infected articles and surfaces; and in the widespread adoption of inoculation of a mild attack of small pox. This in most instances gave almost complete personal protection, usually for the duration of individual life, without the facial disfigurement characteristic of natural small pox; but, unless rigid precautions were taken it became a danger to the public. With the discovery of vaccination, it was no longer justified, even if all possible precautions were taken, for a small proportion of those inoculated died and the risk of infecting others was great; and inoculation, although practised to a diminishing extent for many years after the discovery of vaccination was made definitely illegal in Great Britain in 1840.

B. VACCINATION

The story of the beginning of vaccination has been often told; and it will only be briefly outlined here. It constitutes a supremely important chapter in the history of preventive medicine; and such vaccination may remain unique, unless Calmette's use of mitigated living tubercle bacilli for protecting children against familial infection should be confirmed by experience. With this possible exception, the more recent immunizations secured since Pasteur's pioneer efforts,—for protection against cholera, typhoid fever, diphtheria and perhaps scarlet fever,—have been made with sterilized cultures of the respective micro-organisms of these diseases.

The main points in the history of Jenner's work can

be briefly summarised. They furnish a further example (see page 47) of the value of hypothesis in providing the necessary impetus to exact investigation. Edward Jenner was born in Berkeley in 1749, and his life-work was done in this small town. When aged 21 he became a house pupil of John Hunter, and owed much to his example and criticism. He had previously been the pupil of a surgeon at Godbury since the age of 13; and while there heard a girl make the remark: "I cannot take small pox, for I have had cow pox." He passed on this remark a few years later to Hunter, who wisely advised: "Do not think, but try; be patient, be accurate." On returning to Berkeley, Jenner found that the milkers of the district were generally of opinion that infection with cow pox protected against small pox, and the subject continually occupied his mind. In 1780, not yet having demonstrated the truth of the hypothesis, he revealed his belief confidentially to friends; and between 1788 and 1796 he was making experimental inquiries. In 1798 his famous *Inquiry* was published, containing the proof of the belief popularly entertained. A dairy-maid, Sarah Nelms, scratched her hand, which was subsequently infected with the cow pox from her master's cows. Jenner took some of the vaccine virus from this girl's hand on May 14th, 1796, and vaccinated James Phipps with this matter on his arm. Typical vaccinia followed. On July 1st he was inoculated with variolous matter directly abstracted from a small pox patient. No disease followed. Some months afterwards a repetition of this experiment had the same negative result.

In addition to this direct evidence, Jenner made the following additional observations. His cases were divided into several groups.

a. Cases illustrating protection against Small Pox by Cow-pox

Case I. Joseph M. had cow-pox 1770. Inoculated several times with small-pox 1795. No effect.

Case II. Sarah P. Cow-pox 1765. In 1792 nursed small-pox children and was inoculated in both arms. No effect.

Case III. John P. at age 9 had cow-pox. At age 62 inoculated with small-pox. No effect, except "an efflorescence."

Case IV. Mary B. Cow-pox in 1760. Inoculated with small-pox 1791. No effect.

Case V. Mrs. H. Cow-pox in early life. Inoculated 1778. No effect.

b. Cases of protection against cow-pox by small pox

Case VI. Cow-pox outbreak on Mr. B's farm 1796, five persons. All except dairy-maid had gone through small-pox: of these 2 escaped cow-pox, 2 had a sore on one finger; and the dairy-maid had cow-pox severely.

Case VII. Cow-pox occurred in persons having had small-pox, but much more severe in one member of the family who had not had small-pox.

c. Arm to arm vaccination

Case VIII. William Peed, aged 8 was vaccinated from William Summers March 28th, who had cow-pox.

Case IX, etc. From William Peed 6 persons were vaccinated, and these experiments were continued in series.

Jenner remarks: "These experiments afforded me much satisfaction; they proved that the matter in passing from one human subject to another, through five gradations, lost none of its original properties." The efficacy of the vaccination in some of these cases, and particularly in William Peed, was tested by subsequent unsuccessful inoculation with small pox.

The above account is curtailed; but even so, serves to indicate the thoroughness of Jenner's demonstration of the accuracy of the hypothesis from which he started. The chain of evidence was complete, and his thesis in his own words was placed on a rock "where I knew it would be immovable before I invited the public to take a look at it."

In both Europe and America, notwithstanding much opposition, vaccination was rapidly accepted as an efficient protective against small pox; and it is established and now almost universally admitted that successful vaccination protects entirely from attack by small pox for some years, and mitigates the severity of any attack which may subsequently occur.

CHAPTER XX

The Prevention of Non-specific Infection (Sepsis)

It is probable that in human history non-specific infections, following on wounds, injuries, and parturition, have destroyed more lives than the infectious diseases which are presumably or certainly caused by specific microörganisms. The first impression of incredulity at such a statement will be vastly reduced on consideration of the vast improvement in health and the enormous saving of lives secured through Lister's work. Lister's achievement was in some measure anticipated in mediaeval times. Hippocrates and Galen had taught that suppuration was a normal occurrence in the healing of wounds; and many still living can remember the day when surgeons spoke of "laudable pus." Now suppuration is an index of partial failure in surgery. The old Friar's Balsam, by furnishing a protective film over wounded surfaces, embodied an element of antiseptic precaution. The old idea of treating wounds with boiling oil also seemed to have had behind it the same notion: and the story is well known of how Ambroise Paré (1510–1590) discovered accidentally that wounds not thus treated did equally well, and that ligature of arteries was better than cauterization by a red hot iron. Paracelsus about the same time proclaimed that wounds for the most part would heal if left alone. He added:

> Cautiously the Surgeon must take heed not to remove or to interfere with Nature's balsam, but protect and defend it in its working and in its virtue. . . . . It is the nature of flesh to possess in itself an innate balsam.

But the first clear teaching combating the ancient views as to suppuration appears to have been by Theoderic, born in Italy, A.D. 1208, of whom Dr. C. K. Hindley has written an interesting study ("Aseptic Surgery in the Fourteenth Century," *Nineteenth Century Magazine*, October, 1925). Theoderic advocated immediate closing of the edges of the wound, after applying warm wine, and removing all foreign matter. Theoderic's teaching that suppuration is a complication in a wound was extended by H. de Mandeville, who was bold enough to say that "God did not exhaust all His creative power, when he made Galen." Unfortunately, on his death the new view was forgotten or neglected, and for nearly 600 years suppuration continued its deadly work, until the work of Pasteur and Lister introduced a new era.

The epoch-making work of Lister belongs to the Pasteurian period; and further allusion to it must therefore be postponed; but in this chapter a sketch must be given of a remarkable anticipation of Lister's methods in the care of parturition. Childbearing is a physiological process, which should not come within the range of disease; but in all ages it has been liable to complications dangerous to the life and well-being of mother or infant or both. For ages the care of women in childbirth was undertaken chiefly by women neighbours or midwives, whose only competence was that derived from the mistakes of experience. Ambroise Paré and his pupil Guillimeau introduced some improvements in practice; including version in shoulder presentations. But it was the midwifery forceps which dealt the greatest blow to the prestige of the midwives. The use of these,—first introduced by the Chamberlin family who retained some proprietary rights over them—has doubtless saved many lives and much suffering; but we are now learning that their unwise and hurried use may be the cause of serious mischief to maternal tissues and of sepsis, and may also produce tentorial tearing and other cranial injuries in the infant. The historic nose of Tristam Shandy was disfigured by the use of forceps. It may be noted that in the seventeenth century Harvey practised as a man-midwife and helped to rescue English midwifery from its age of darkness. He also denounced the meddlesome midwifery of his time. The advance of midwifery led to the establishment of Lying-in Hospitals for the poor. For many years "Puerperal fever"—which had been first named and described by Thomas Willis (1621–1675)—was their bane; but since the introduction of antiseptics and the application of the principles of modern scientific midwifery, the maternal mortality in these institutions—if all classes of cases are included—has been much lower than is yet experienced in private practice.

The history of enlightenment as to puerperal sepsis is instructive, so slowly in the past have exact observation and careful inferences from facts been accepted by generations of physicians who were obsessed by fixed dogmas. Four names are specially worthy of remembrance,—White of Manchester, Gordon of Aberdeen, Oliver Wendell Holmes of Boston, Massachusetts, and Semmelweis of Vienna and Budapest,—but not one of them succeeded in convincing the mass of the medical profession, until the greater work of Pasteur and Lister finally dispersed the old-time prejudices.

Dr. Chas. White, F.R.S., writing in 1773, in his *Management of Pregnancy and Lying-in Women* made the following enlightened statement:

> As the puerperal fever does not appear till after delivery, and so neither does absorption of matter from an abscess till it is opened and the air have access, we may, I think, with a good deal of certainty, conclude that the absorption of matter is the immediate cause of the puerperal fever, as well as that consequent upon abscesses and ulcers.

In this remark he anticipated Sir James Simpson's well-known essay on the close analogy between the fever following sugrical operations and that occurring in lying-in women. (For further particulars see Dr. C. Cullingworth's brochure, 1904, on "C. White, A great provincial surgeon and obstetrician of the eighteenth century".)

The superiority of the view quoted above over that of Semmelweis consisted in the fact that it explains cases arising from self-infection (autochthonous) as well as cases in which infection is introduced by contamination from without.

Reference should be made also to Dr. A. Gordon of Aberdeen, who was quoted by O. W. Holmes. He concluded that "the cause of this disease (puerperal fever) was a specific contagion or infection, I have unquestionable proof . . . . as readily communicable as the infection of small-pox or measles."

Dr. Gordon in his pamphlet wrote: "it is a disagreeable declaration for me to mention that I myself was the means of carrying the infection to a great number of women;" and he cited other cases in the practice of midwives and of other doctors. In the class-room of the Professor of Midwifery in the University of Aberdeen is an inscription stating that Gordon "first demonstrated the infectious nature of puerperal fever, 1795."

Not the smallest claim of Oliver Wendell Holmes (1809–1894) to remembrance consists in his impressive and brave writing on this subject. His first essay on "The Contagiousness of Puerperal Fever" was published in 1843, six or seven years before any of Semmelweis' results were made public. This essay went to establish the thesis that puerperal fever is "communicated from one person to another, both directly and indirectly." He brushed aside negative facts, reminding his readers: "children that walk in calico before open fires are not always burnt to death," and such facts are not to be used as arguments against woollen frocks and high fenders. Holmes's main conclusion was that puerperal fever is frequently carried from patient to patient by physicians and nurses. He limited his view of the subject to the passage of infection from previous cases. He did not contend as to the mode of infection, but contented himself with the statement of the well-known fact that "contagious diseases frequently spare those who appear to be fully submitted to their influence." He held to the view that apart from the infection, the disease might be modified by causes other than contagion, and referred also to "the undoubted fact that within the walls of lying-in hospitals there is often generated a miasm, palpable as the chlorine used to destroy it, tenacious as in some cases almost to defy extirpation, deadly in some institutions as the plague."

In subsequent editions of Holmes's essay, he defended himself most cogently against those opposing his views. Perhaps the most strongly worded expression of disbelief came from Dr. C. L. Meigs (1797–1869),[1] who ridiculed Holmes's deductions as the "jejune and fizzenless vaporings of sophomore writers," and interpreted cases of puerperal fever as

[1] Quoted in Dr. Whitridge Williams' *A Sketch of the History of Obstetrics in the United States* (1903).

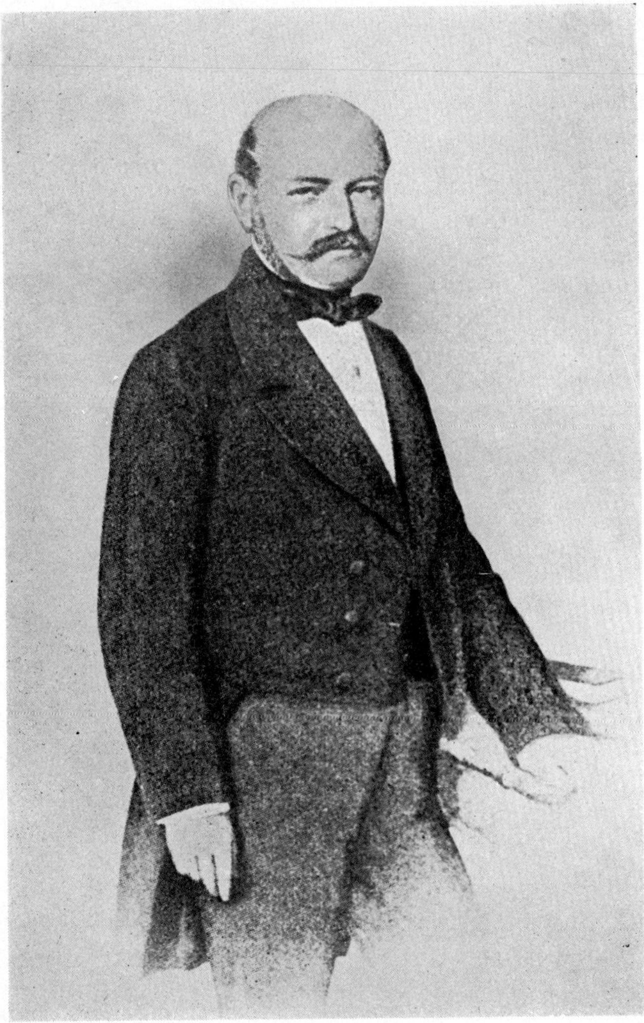

Ignatz Philipp Semmelweis (1818–1865)

due to "accident or Providence," or perhaps to "a contagion on which I cannot form any clear idea, at least as to this particular malady."

In the final monograph which Holmes wrote in 1855, entitled *Puerperal Fever as a Private Pestilence* he was able to quote Semmelweis's experience in support, and we may quote in conclusion a sentiment written by Holmes later in his life:

> By the permission of Providence I held up to the professional public the damnable facts connected with the conveyance of poison from one young mother's chamber to another's—for doing which humble service I desire to be thankful that I have lived, though nothing else good should ever come to my life.

To Ignaz Phillip Semmelweis (1818–1865) belongs the supreme credit of devising measures for preventing puerperal sepsis, and of proving their efficacy in practice. In this respect Semmelweis—although Lister when in 1865 he first applied the antiseptic principle to wounds knew nothing of Semmelweis's work—was a forerunner of Listerism, teaching its application in the realm of midwifery. He happened on the truth before his time, and the stress of his advocacy of it brought this unstable genius to insanity. It should be added at once that while Holmes was concerned with the transmission of infection from patient to patient, Semmelweis laid chief stress on infective material from dead bodies.

Semmelweis was a Magyar, born in Budapest, and as a student in Vienna became an assistant in the

1st obstetric ward of the Allgemeines Krankenhaus. This ward was so notorious for its high mortality in lying-in cases, that women begged in tears not to be admitted to it. Under Rokitansky it fell to Semmelweis to make many autopsies on dead parturient women. His active mind at once concentrated on this question. Starting from the assumption that "pregnancy was not a nine-months' disease," he examined the experience of the two divisions of the maternity clinic, of which the first was served by medical students, the second by midwives. In the first puerperal infection was rife, in the second exceptional. The general conditions of the two were identical, except that, owing to its greater popularity, there was more crowding in the second division. The cases of puerperal disease could scarcely be due to epidemic influences; for if so why should one of the two clinics under the same roof be saved? Furthermore, it was noteworthy that women surprised by labour in the streets escaped the infection, to whichever division they were admitted. On March 20th, 1847, on returning to Vienna after a short holiday, Semmelweis was present at the autopsy of a friend who had died from lymphangitis, phlebitis and peritonitis, following a prick on the finger at an autopsy; and it flashed across his mind that as the post mortem findings in the two instances were similar if not identical, the puerperal women and Kolletschka alike had died from septic infection.

A new regulation was at once made for the students.

Before touching a woman (hitherto they had come straight from dissecting rooms without precautions) they must wash their hands in a solution of chloride of lime. Thus as one has put it, a chunk of chloride of lime upset a basketful of theories. The special incidence of puerperal sepsis on the wards served by medical students at once ceased.

Semmelweis in 1860 said "Puerperal fever is not a contagious disease, but it is conveyable from a sick to a sound puerpera by means of decomposed organic material." Thus he regarded puerperal fever as a form of pyoemia, capable of being produced by a disease which is not puerperal fever.

We now know that puerperal sepsis may be caused by autogenic poisoning, especially by haemolytic streptococci, but that more often it is due to infection conveyed from patient to patient, or to infection derived from other septic sources. Indeed all those whose contributions to this subject have been outlined, had contributed portions of the truth, and the synthesis of these reveals the full possibilities of prevention.

Some of the chief professors in Vienna accepted Semmelweis's conclusion, and Hebra linked Semmelweis's name with that of Edward Jenner, and entrusted his own wife to Semmelweis's care!

But others fiercely opposed Semmelweis, and at the age of 31 he was practically driven out of Vienna (see Sir W. Sinclair's *Life of Semmelweis*, 1909). In Budapest he had similar obstruction to meet. He became obsessed with the supreme importance of the precautions, which on every hand were neglected, as was also his teaching, by Virchow among others. His language in his writings became more and more emphatic. He inveighed against the discussion of epidemic influences "while the examining finger and the operating hand committed murder." He grew bitter and irritable. His writings became a "burning lash and a flaming sword." Writing to Scanzoni he said:

> If . . . . without controverting my teachings, or giving reasons for assuming them erroneous, you continue to teach your students the doctrine of epidemic puerperal fever, I denounce you before God and the world as a murderer, and the history of Puerperal Fever, will not do you an injustice when, for the service of having been the first to oppose my life-saving *Lehre*, it perpetuates your name as a medical Nero.

He became known as the Hungarian crank, and in 1865, when forty-seven years old he was removed to a lunatic asylum.

He was found to have a wound on his finger, the result of his last gynoecological operation. He quickly developed pyaemia, and thus died of the disease, the way to prevent which, in women in childbirth, he had demonstrated,—alas! some decades before the elementary precautions taught by him began to be taken. How many physicians have died of the diseases which they have specially studied? Laennec died of phthisis, Charles Murchison of cardiac disease occurring after two attacks of typhus.

The story of the prevention of sepsis is a great chapter in the history of preventive medicine. It is a chapter the greater part of which *in practice* still remains to be written. The sketch given in the preceding pages shews great potentialities, but unhappily puerperal septis remains unnecessarily frequent. The study of Lister's great work cannot be told in this volume. By antiseptic and aseptic surgery, with the aid of modern anaesthesia, life has been prolonged and saved, sickness and invalidity have been reduced, and the standard of human life and happiness have been almost incredibly improved. But the possibilities of removal of sepsis have not yet been exhausted; and in connection with tonsillar and adenoid work, with dental treatment, with the discovery of focal infections, there still stretch before us ranges of curative and preventive treatment not hitherto attained.

CHAPTER XXI

Food and Drink in Relation to Health

Food and Drink are prime necessaries of life, and the struggle to obtain them has been a chief factor in determining the course of human history. Whoever first applied fire to the cooking of food, took a momentous step out of barbarism; and there can be little doubt that the devotion for many ages of the Chinese to tea-drinking has saved them from many devastating epidemics.

The lack of food on a large scale, constituting Famine, has made landmarks in human history. Almost always famine has been accompanied or followed by pestilence, especially by cholera and typhus; and in the past the privation of food was regarded as directly responsible for the infection as well as for lowering resistance to disease. We now know that, as in the instance of the Potato Famine in Ireland in the year 1846, famines were responsible for pestilence largely if not chiefly because they necessitated wide wanderings of destitute people, many of whom were incubating disease, in search of nourishment (see page 131). The occurrence of widespread destitution, amounting almost to famine, has necessitated compulsory provision for the starving; and we owe the genesis of the English system of poor-law relief in Elizabethan days to this motive power. In the incidence of its expense and in its effect poor-law relief constitutes a national system of insurance against starvation (page 117).

More rapid means of communication, both between parts of the same country and between different countries, have greatly reduced the possibilities of famine, and have permitted the growth of a population many times as great in countries which are chiefly industrial than would have otherwise been possible in the present stage of development of farming and gardening. Hence the steam engine and more recently the gas engine and the internal-combustion engine have been important factors in preventive medicine. The reduction of length of sea voyages has been a supremely important factor in increasing food supplies as well as in causing the practical cessation of scurvy.

This disease in past centuries has been a terrible cause of sickness and death both on land and sea, and particularly to sailors, to soldiers in campaigns, to the inhabitants of beleagured cities, and to those in public institutions whether prisons or workhouses. On land it became rare long before it disappeared from our naval and mercantile marine; and in the Great War 1914–18 sporadic cases occurred in workhouses when potatoes were unobtainable. The introduction of the potato and the increase in the use of other fresh vegetable food have been the chief factors in the disappearance of scurvy in civilian experience. The potato was introduced from America into both Spain and England between 1560 and 1570; and was brought by Raleigh in 1585 from North Carolina and Virginia, and cultivated on his estates near Cork.

The dependence of scurvy on the lack of fresh food was well known for many years before action was taken to prevent its occurrence on board ship. The British Navy was more than once rendered almost impotent for service by the ravages of scurvy. Admiral Anson in his celebrated voyage of 1740–2 lost in ten months nearly two-thirds of his crew of 961 men, chiefly from scurvy. At an earlier date Sir Richard Hawkins, a great Elizabethan navigator, said that in 20 years he had known of 10,000 seamen having perished by scurvy alone; and Blane told an equally unfavorable story so late as 1780. The dietary on board a ship of war, as Dr. W. A. Guy reminds us (*Public Health: A Popular Introduction*, 1870), often consisted in pre-reform days of beef badly salted, and sometimes so rotten that, before boiling it, it was necessary to tie it round with cords; biscuits mouldy and full of weevils or maggots; and puddings of salt, suet, and flour. In Anson's voyage many difficulties were experienced, from which Captain Cook escaped in his first voyage in 1772, with which Anson's experience is often contrasted. Nevertheless, Captain Cook's experience was most striking. Out of a crew of 118, and during an absence from England of 3 years and 18 days, Captain Cook, in a voyage round the world, lost only 4 men, three by accident and one from phthisis. Instances might be multiplied. Guy illustrates the contrast between the adoption of anti-scorbutic prophylaxis and its absence by the fact that in 1800 the Channel Fleet kept the sea for four months without one vessel being in port, and brought back only 16 patients for hospital; while only twenty years earlier, the same fleet was so overrun with scurvy and fever as to be unable to keep the sea for ten weeks together; and in many years national safety was endangered by the scorbutic condition of the sailors in the Navy.

The pitiful condition of the sailors occupied much thought. Mr. S. Sutton, like many others, considered the chief enemy to be the terribly defective ventilation in the ships; and backed by Dr. Richard Mead in 1749 he succeeded in getting his system of ventilation of holds tried. Dr. Hales made attempts to the same end. It may be added that in Mead's description of Sutton's ventilator,—in a paper to the Royal Society—he speaks of the beneficial effect of oranges. He also makes mention of the recommendation of the Royal College of Physicians to the Lords of the Admiralty that wine-vinegar should be supplied to every ship. "This qualifies the salt of the food, and makes some amends for the want of sub-acid fruits." Mead also alluded to the value of vegetable foods; but, like Sutton, he attached chief importance to bad air in the causation of scurvy.

Captain Cook's paper describing his successful voyage was read to the Royal Society on 30th November, 1776, and the Copley Medal of the Society was awarded to him, He is reported to have uttered a wise dictum: "Precautions are always blamed; whenever they are successful, they are said to be unnecessary." He laid more stress on general hygiene than on the use of anti-scorbutics, and expressed a guarded view on the value of the "rob of oranges and lemons proposed by Lind for use at sea."

But the value of anti-scorbutic foods in the prevention of scurvy had been known long before Captain Cook's successful circum-navigation of the world. The Dutch as far back as 1564 recognized the value of fresh fruit and vegetables for the prevention and cure of scurvy. In 1601 Purchas (quoted by Simon) shewed the virtue of lemon-juice against scurvy as evidenced in the first voyage made for the East India Company in 1600; and John Woodall, surgeon-general to the East India Company, in "The Surgeon's Mate," 1617, advised lemon-juice both for prophylaxis and treatment.

It is to Dr. James Lind (*Treatise on the Scurvy*, 1st edition, 1754) that the chief credit is due for describing scurvy accurately, and for stating clearly what was required for its practical prevention. Before him varied conditions had been described as scorbutic, and Dr. Gideon Harvey, Charles II's physician, made over 20 species of scurvy. Any condition of the skin not readily yielding to treatment, including itch, was called scorbutic. Lind himself was not free from the medical obsessions of his period. He (on page 183, 2nd edition) says:

> A most powerful and principal cause of scurvy and indeed of many other maladies, is the moisture of the air, and consequently the dampness of their (sailors') lodging; especially during a long continuance of thick close weather, or a stormy and rainy season.

But he is absolutely definite in his main practical statement:

> Experience sufficiently proves that as greens or vegetables, with ripe fruits, are the best remedies for it, so they prove the most effectual preservatives against it.

Lind entered the naval service in 1739 at the age of 23, serving until 1748. He became physician to the Haslar Naval Hospital from 1758–1783. According to Dr. R. Stockman (*Edinburgh Medical Journal*, June, 1926), 1,146 scorbutic patients were admitted to Haslar in his first year, one-fifth of the total admissions; and during the seven years of the war with France and Spain he usually had 300 to 400 cases of scurvy under his daily charge. By one of his contemporaries Lind has been called a "Marine Hippocrates," and his pioneer work places him high up in the rank of his contemporaries in preventive medicine; only excelled among them in beneficent influence on the welfare of mankind by William Jenner and John Howard.

For convenience of reference, let me place here the dates of birth and death of the chief pioneers of hygiene in this eventful period:

Richard Mead	1673–1754
John Pringle	1707–1782
James Lind	1716–1794
Gilbert Blane	1749–1834
Edward Jenner	1740–1823
John Howard	1726–1790

But although Lind had clearly shewn in 1754 the action needed to suppress scurvy, and similar but less exact and complete knowledge had been published in English in 1617, a further latent period of forty-one years elapsed before Lind's teaching was applied in practice; and then it was Dr. afterwards Sir Gilbert Blane on his appointment on the Navy Medical Board of the Admiralty, who in 1795 forced through the necessary reform. Earlier experience gained as physician to the Fleet led him in 1781 to lay a memorial before the Board of Admiralty recommending several reforms, including a supply of lemon juice to prevent and cure scurvy. His recommendations had fallen on deaf ears. Lemon juice was made a compulsory ration to the British Navy in 1795. Prior to this Blane had arranged experimental trials of lemon juice as remedy and prophylactic. In 1794 a small East Indian squadron was equipped with an adequate supply. The squadron without touching port arrived at the end of twenty-three days in

Madras without a case of scurvy, and trial in the Channel Fleet was equally successful. Many commanders had anticipated the Admiralty's order of 1795, and the new compulsory provision was dramatically successful. Trotter, writing in 1803, said: "A case of scurvy requiring to be sent to hospital has not come under my observation since 1795;" and Blane in 1813 stated that scurvy was now as rare at sea as on land.

In 1780 on a ten weeks' cruise the Channel Fleet was over-run with scurvy; in 1800, during a cruise of four months, not a single case occurred. The successes of Nelson and Collingwood in their naval surveillance over France's ships were made possible by the compulsory measures against scurvy, and Lind should be remembered not only as a great pioneer in the application of preventive medicine, but also as greatly contributing to the prospects of national success in the great anti-Napoleonic struggle. In a later generation Dr. Takaki was similarly successful in initiating measures for ridding the Japanese Navy of beri-beri (p. 198).

A compulsory measure backed by the necessary discipline secured the abolition of a dietetic disease; and this is noteworthy as the first instance on record of compulsion in a matter of food and drink being imposed on a large section of the entire community. Two Acts of Parliament, in 1844 and 1847, were required before complete compulsion on similar lines was adopted in the mercantile marine. It appears to be the case that disregard by the medical profession and the obsession of medical teachers by their own theories were more responsible for this delay than official inaction. The ration at one time has been lime juice instead of lemon juice; but lime juice is less effective than lemon juice.

Beri-beri. We may refer here to another disease which like scurvy is a deficiency disease. The prevention of beri-beri is one of the chief triumphs of Japan, and it is convenient to mention it here, although it was not until 1880 that Dr. Takaki, afterwards Surgeon-General Takaki, who had just returned from St. Thomas's Hospital, London, where he had been a medical student, began to investigate the incidence of this disease. He found a great disproportion between the number of cases on board ship and in barracks, this being associated with a deficiency of nitrogenous food in the navy. In 1883 the war-ship Ruyajo went on a voyage of 271 days to New Zealand and South America, and over 100 cases of beri-beri occurred among the 350 persons on board. Another ship, the Tarkula, was then sent exactly on the same course, and under the same conditions, so far as these could be duplicated, except that a new diet scale was arranged which avoided an excess of rice. On this trip only 16 cases of beri-beri occurred. The following figures shew the incidence of beri-beri per 100 of Force in the Japanese Navy in the years during which great reforms were instituted. These included a more liberal supply of nitrogenous food, much less rice, and general hygienic improvements.

1878	32.8
1879	38.0
1884	12.4
1888	0.00
1889	0.03

During the subsequent naval war with Russia no case occurred in a floating force of over 25,000. The Japanese Army, with medical advisers of German training, was reluctant to adopt the naval reforms, and in the Russian war it is stated that nearly one half of the Army sickness was caused by kakki (beri-beri). Further particulars are given in Dr. L. L. Seaman's *The Real Triumph of Japan*, 1906.

The more recent discoveries in dietetics, and especially those concerned with deficiency diseases and the rôle of vitamins in the prevention of disease are within the recent knowledge of most of us, and are omitted from discussion here. Similarly the new knowledge as to the prevention of goitre by the administration of iodine can only be mentioned.

Alcohol. It is with regret that I find myself unable to devote a separate chapter to the story of alcoholic control as bearing on public health progress. The history of the eighteenth and nineteenth century in England, as well as in America—and to some extent in other countries—illustrates increasing realisation of the urgent need for some measure of control over the sale of alcoholic drinks. Scurvy (page 196) forms a striking instance of compulsory addition to human dietary (in the naval and mercantile marine). But alcohol affords a scarcely less striking and an even more important instance of the enforcement of regulations against the most eagerly desired drinks of mankind. These regulations historically have been successful, in so far as they embodied an overwhelming educated public opinion, in reducing the consumption of alcoholic drinks, and in thus paralysing one of the chief enemies of preventive medicine.

Food poisoning and sophistication. Early sanitary action was largely concerned with the prevention of sale of food unfit for human consumption. The ancient Jewish enactments regarding meat were extremely strict; and Kosher meat still has undergone much more rigid inspection with some measure of rejection than is likely to be practised for the bulk of Gentile meat, so long as small private slaughter-houses are allowed to continue. The danger of consumption of beef and pork infected with either the cysticercus of the tape-worm, or with trichinæ is well known; such meat is now seldom seen.

The relation of infection of milk to the production of epidemics of scarlet fever, typhoid fever, diphtheria, and sore throats, has already been indicated (p. 140). There is no doubt also that a considerable share of the tuberculosis of joints and glands in children is due to the drinking of uncooked milk from tuberculous cows.

The common practice of pasteurization or boiling of milk and the additional care now taken in the production and sale of milk have greatly reduced these risks.

The sophistication of many articles of food has been commonly practised. It goes back to ancient times. Pliny alludes to the frauds practised by bakers; and both in ancient Athens and Rome wine was much tampered with. Bread was the subject of legal regulation in England as early as the reign of King John, the chief object being to limit the profit of the baker. In 1582 provisions were inserted against the adulteration of meal, as well as against the sale of "mesell pork," etc., punishment being inflicted of a fine, or the pillory, or for a third or fourth offence that the offender shall "forswere the towne." Mineral substances such as alum were added to conceal the use of inferior flour.

In France in 1382 there were ordinances against the use of damaged flour, the substitution of other materials for corn, or light weight. In Germany there were similar regulations, of which particulars are given in Blyth's *Foods*, (4th edition, 1896).

In the early part of the 19th century there was much activity against adulteration of foods; and in most civilized countries there are now public analysts and food inspectors to secure the examination of suspected foods, and the prosecution of offenders.

From the standpoint of health the sophistication of milk is the most important of all adulterations. It is the chief food of infants and young children; and the addition of water and the abstraction of cream both imply deprivation to the extent of the deterioration of an essential element in nutrition.

Next to this comes the protection against chemical preservatives in foods. Boric acid and other preservatives in the past have been added to so many foods that although the amount in any one article may not be injurious the cumulative effect of preservatives is serious. This is now a decreasing evil.

CHAPTER XXII

Infantile Hygiene

It will have been seen in preceding chapters that in actual experience preventive medicine is largely concerned with the treatment of already established disease with the aim of (*a*) terminating it as speedily as possible, (*b*) preventing the occurrence of the personal familial and social sequelae which so commonly haunt the footsteps of illness, and (*c*) securing the adoption of advice and action on it which will prevent the operation of the recurring causes of illness.

Thus in childhood rickets is treated and its further progress stayed; adenoids and tonsillar troubles are treated, and thus mouth-breathing, deafness and artificial stupidity are abated or ended; acute rheumatic conditions are placed under skilled care and cardiac therapeutics and restoration of physical efficiency are made possible. So also in tuberculosis, the treatment of the individual patient often leads to his restoration; even if not, after intelligent, sympathetic and hygienic treatment, the patient is not likely to continue to be a source of danger to those about him, and especially to children.

Syphilis, perhaps more than any other disease, illustrates the supremely high value of treatment as a means of prevention. A single dose of arseno-benzol diminishes and may abolish the infectivity of superficial lesions of this disease; and systematic treatment entirely destroys the infectivity of syphilis by curing the patient. Evidently then treatment must always hold a high place in the practice of preventive medicine.

But the ultimate aim and in some measure the immediately practicable objective of preventive medicine, is to obviate the need for treatment by the application of the known laws of hygiene; and the period of life in which this is especially possible is in the antenatal and post-natal period of an infant's life. I can only indicate here some of the earlier struggles towards this idea, especially in regard to food, the prime need of life.

The gross measure of failure of hygiene is the occurrence of an excessive number of deaths of infants. Some of this excessive mortality in the past has been intentional; the exposures of infants on the Ganges and in ancient Greece are instances of this; as is also the vast amount of abortion running through the ages.

Prior to 1837 when registration of births and deaths became obligatory in England, exact statistical data were lacking; but there is no doubt that both in England and in other countries the rate of infant mortality was often appallingly high. The high birth-rate was counteracted by the high death-rate; and this largely explained the low rate of increase of population prior to the eighteenth century. Privation often so general as to constitute famine, neglect, especially the neglect associated with gin drinking and drunkenness, and gross ignorance of methods of feeding all from time to time were at work. In the first half of the eighteenth century it is probable that three-fourths of the infants born died before reaching the age of five years, the proportion dying being about two-fifths of those born in the latter part of that century. In England the rate of infant mortality i. e., mortality under one year per 1,000 births stated in quinquennial periods beginning with 1841–1845, and ending with 1896–1900 was as follows: 148, 157, 156, 152, 151, 157, 153, 145, 139, 145, 151, 156. These figures represented a great improvement on earlier experience; which in large measure is explained by the fact that small-pox had ceased to be a large factor in causing deaths in early life; but no evidence of continuing improvement is displayed in them. It must be assumed, therefore, that during these fifty-five years the main causes of mortality in infants varied but little from one quinquennium to another.

A very different story is seen in the experience of the quinquennial periods 1901–1905 to 1921–1925: 138, 117, 110, 90, 76. Evidently some new factors favourably influencing the vitality of infants have come into play, among which improved sanitation, domestic and communal, and more intelligent care of infants, including greater personal cleanliness and more satisfactory methods of feeding infants may be specially mentioned. Not much attention was paid to the medical care of infants prior to the 18th century. Even in well-to-do households with large families the number surviving beyond childhood was relatively small. Glisson's remarkable work on rickets was printed in 1650, and in 1669 John Magow wrote on the same subject. In the eighteenth century several guides to the management of children appeared.

Dr. William Cadogan published an "Essay on Nursing" in 1747, intended for the guidance of the Governors of the Foundling Hospital, in which he advised fresh air and proper exercise and four-hourly intervals of feeding.

In 1769 Dr. George Armstrong started a Dispensary in London for the relief of the infant poor. It was the first devoted solely to the relief of children. He wrote an account of the diseases most incident to children.

In 1821 Dr. J. Bunnell Davis edited the *Annals of the Universal Dispensary for Children* which had recently been opened for children under twelve; and appended to this report "a cursory inquiry into some of the principal causes of mortality among children, with a view to assist in ameliorating the state of the rising generation." He stated that in 1815 in London within the Bills of Mortality there were recorded 19,560 deaths at all ages, of which over one-third occurred at ages under five.

The importance of breast feeding was strongly urged by Dr. Michael Underwood, who published *A Treatise on the Diseases of Children* in 1784. In this he deprecated the tendency to exaggerate dentition as a disease of children, and protested against Dr. Arbuthnot's statement that one child in ten is supposed to sink under it. He also accused Dr. Armstrong of too much complacency towards tyrant fashion in favouring artificial feeding of infants. "Though apparently an advocate for suckling, he has laboured for arguments to apologize for the spoon and the boat in too many instances."

The modern methods of feeding infants when their mothers are unable or unwilling to suckle, are of comparatively recent date. In the past the choice lay between a wet nurse and "dry nursing." Against the too free use of wet nurses, writers in many ages have inveighed. Tacitus complained that the Roman matrons had begun to entrust their infants to Greek slave girls.

Luigi Tansillo, born in 1510 and therefore a contemporary of Ariosto and Tasso, published a long Italian poem entitled "The Nurse," which was translated into English verse by W. Roscoe (father of the distinguished chemist) in 1800. The main burden of this poem is an exhortation to mothers not to neglect their natural duty. Some stanzas may be quoted:

> What! could she, as her own existence dear,
> Nine tedious months her tender burthen bear,
> Yet when at length it smiled upon the day,
> To hireling hands its helpless frame convey?
>
> . . . .
>
> Does no remorse, ye fair, your bosoms gnaw,
> Rebellious to affection's primal law?
>
> . . . .

Spontaneous then supply the milky spring;
The only voluntary boon ye bring.

. . . .

Say, can ye choose a nurse from broad St. Giles?
Heedless what venom taints the stream she gives,
So your stall'd offspring vegetates and lives.

Somewhat later (1584) appeared a Latin poem entitled "Poedotrophia: or the Art of Nursing and Rearing Children," of which Dr. H. W. Tyler published an English translation in 1787.

There is on page 98 an interesting allusion to the protracted suckling which still persists in some countries:

She should not of her pleasing duty tire
Nor from the boy
Withdraw the breast; nor other cares employ
Her heart, and fostering hand, till twice the sun
His annual journey round the globe had run.

The wide use of wet nurses led to much incidental mischief. (See Dr. Forsyth's "The History of Infant Feeding from Elizabethan Times," *Proc. Roy. Soc. of Med.*, Vol. IV, 1911, p. 114.) In Elizabethan days, as in the Victorian period before the passing of the Infant Life Protection Act in 1872, the baby-farmers were plying their evil trade; and illegitimacy became a profitable undertaking, because of the prospective gain of the mother as a wet nurse.

Dry nursing is seldom mentioned in the writings on children prior to the eighteenth century. Suckling was usually protracted; and a common rule was that a child should not be weaned before it had all its teeth. In the Georgian period, the spoon and the boat were the chief means for artificial feeding of infants; but Dr. Hugh Smith, *Letters to Married Women*, 1784, 3rd edition, gained much reputation by his invention of an urn-like pot, with a mouth resembling a nipple. Prior to this a polished cow's horn was often used, its small end being perforated, and two pieces of parchment attached and sewn together, so that milk could be sucked through between the stitches. Dr. Smith's figures of child mortality derived from the London Bills of Mortality for 1762–1771 may be quoted at this point. The burials of children under five to registered births was 623 per 1,000, and of children under two to registered births was 490 per 1,000.

Water-pap—bread soaked in water—was commonly used to supplement cow's milk. Against cow's milk there were strong prejudices. Dr. Underwood, already quoted, urged the importance of boiling milk, and suggested the use of barley-water as a diluent. He expressed wonder that the "custom of stuffing new-born infants with bread could become so universal."

Foundling Hospitals, it is well known, had an appalling mortality. The infant is the greatest of individualists, and when a number of infants are crowded together, diarrhoeal and other infections speedily show the folly of such aggregation. Malthus himself expressed the view that no more effective means of arresting the growth of population could be found than to multiply institutions for receiving new-born infants.

During the nineteenth century it appears to have been taken for granted that for a considerable proportion of infants "dry nursing" was necessary; and much ingenuity was displayed in improving feeding bottles. The long tubed feeding bottle of modern times, with its constant tendency to become foul, has only in the last few years been abolished from the nursery; a host of patent infants' food, intended as substitutes for cow's milk, or to supplement it, have been sold very largely. These foods whether they contained milk or not were prepared in a condensed or desiccated condition. The evils of sweetened condensed milk gradually became realised, and unsweetened condensed milk has now been largely superseded by desiccated whole milk, on which many infants thrive well, if orange juice or some other anti-scorbutic fruit juice is also given. Of the various patent farinaceous or malted foods, it may be generally asserted that they should only be given in strictly defined circumstances. Some of the worst cases of scurvy-rickets (Barlow's disease) have occurred during their administration.

Happily there is a great return to breast-feeding. At an early stage of the modern movement for child welfare, Milk Depots and other centres for distributing cow's milk for infants were unduly prominent; and there was real fear that in the advice given by health visitors, the precautions of dry nursing or artificial feeding should be emphasised in such a way as to ignore the greater problem, how could the health visitor be utilised so as to obviate the need for such artificial feeding.

The Prevention of Rickets. Reference has been made to Glisson, who wrote the first systematic treatise on Rickets. This disease is very common in Great Britain; it is also extremely common among the town-dwellers in the United States, who live in unfavourable quarters, especially it is said in Italians and in Negroes.

It is said to have been almost unknown before people congregated in towns; but this is doubtful. It must be remembered that in the rural parts of England and America, and even in the East, children may be kept indoors away from the beneficent influence of sunshine.

But although still a serious source of illness and death, Rickets is rapidly decreasing in prevalence. Bandy legs and pigeon-shaped chests are much less common than in the past; and it is the less extreme results of Rickets which are now seen. Chief credit in bringing about this change must be given to the increased care of infancy during the present century.

The story of the gradual increasing realisation of the seriousness of Rickets in lowering national health cannot be detailed here for lack of space; but a few points need to be specially noted. Its continued importance as an enemy to child health and as a source of extreme danger to childbearing women is even yet inadequately recognised. It is a very common disease, and we know that it greatly increases the danger from other diseases to which children are liable. Whooping Cough, Measles and Diarrhoea are especially fatal in rickety children; and the prevention of rickets will mean the saving of thousands of children whose lives are now sacrificed to these diseases. Rickets is the cause not only of pelvic but also of spinal and limb deformation, and it is generally associated with a low average weight and height for any given age, and with impaired intellectual development. The exact connection between Rickets and the occurrence of excessive catarrhs followed by adenoids is perhaps doubtful; but there is no question that the sunlight and cod liver oil, which prevent rickets, even in scantily fed children, will also greatly reduce the occurrence of catarrhs. This is not the complete story of the mischief wrought by Rickets. Rickets is the chief cause of pelvic contraction and deformity, and of complicated and difficult parturition, often necessitating operative aid or even caesarean section.

The prevention of the excessive mortality in childbirth resulting from rachitic deformity of the pelvis should be begun 20 or 30 years earlier, immediately after the birth of the future mother. It is within the range of preventive medicine to prevent entirely rachitic pelvic deformities and thus greatly reduce puerperal mortality in the future.

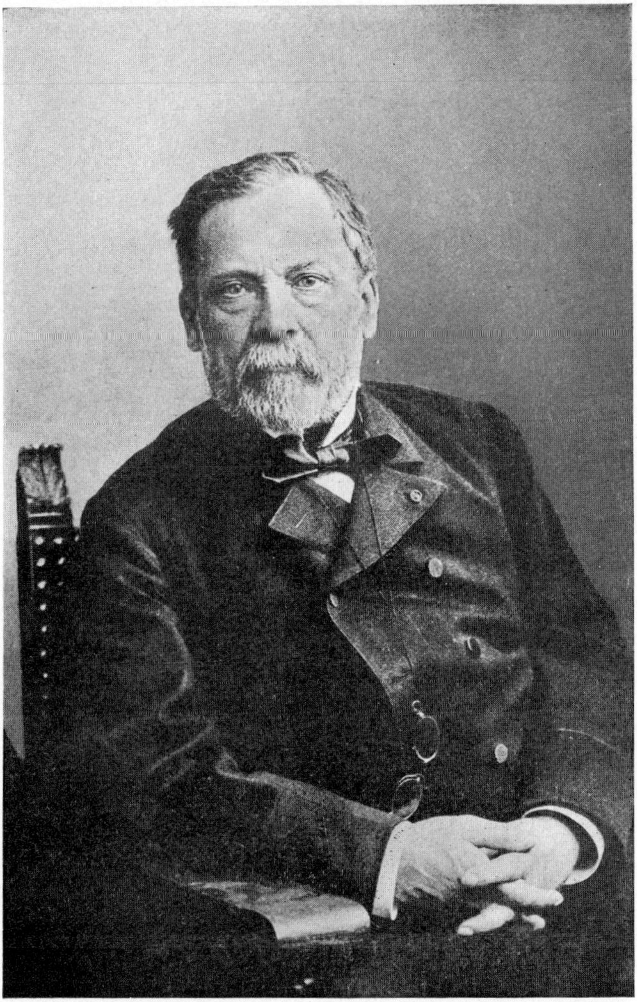

Louis Pasteur (1822–1895)

CHAPTER XXIII

Modern Preventive Medicine

Our sketch of the beginnings and progress of preventive medicine must stop at the stage now reached. Although we have not consistently followed this plan, the sketch as outlined in the preceding chapters has dealt chiefly with the pre-Pasteurian period of medicine. This plan has been deliberately followed, for two reasons. In the first place the more recent history of preventive medicine is relatively familiar, although a second volume in this series in which it is proposed to deal more fully with the last seventy years will tell a fascinating story. In the second place, it is of prime importance that we should all know the pit out of which, with much vicarious suffering, much stumbling in effort, many mistakes, terrible practical errors, we have been digged. Indeed, we may go further, and assert that the value of what we now possess can only be fully appreciated, and utilised by aid of the search light which study of the beginings of things gives us.

In the following paragraphs a few of the outstanding discoveries in preventive medicine during the last seventy years may, in conclusion, be indicated.

Louis Pasteur (1822–1895), a chemist, first discovered that various fermentations, lactic, acetic, etc., were caused by microörganisms, obtaining access to the fermenting liquid from the air.

Schwann in the same year ascertained that meat only became putrid when organisms get into it. From the discovery of the cause of fermentation Pasteur set out to discover the microörganisms which he was confident caused disease. Into his investigations on pebrine (silkworm disease), anthrax, fowl cholera, we cannot enter here; but Pasteur started a new era in investigation, which has been of inestimable benefit to mankind.

Its greatest immediate result was that it inspired Joseph Lister (1827–1913) to initiate antiseptic surgery; and it would be impossible to exaggerate the value of this discovery in saving life, in diminishing suffering, and in increasing the physical efficiency of mankind.

Next among the giants of this period came Robert Koch (1843–1910), who made bacteriology a practical art by devising methods of growing cultures in solid media. He was greatly aided by the use of the anilin stains for staining bacteria, which Weigert had introduced in 1871–1874. Koch's name will always be remembered in connection with his completion of Pasteur's work on anthrax, his discovery of the cholera vibrio, his investigations on typhoid fever, and above all by his discovery of the tubercle bacillus.

Many other discoveries followed in rapid succession. The following is a very incomplete list:

1882—Glanders bacillus discovered by Loeffler.
1882—Tubercle bacillus (Koch).
1883—The vibrio of cholera (Koch).

1884—The tetanus bacillus (Nicolauer).
1887—Micrococcus melitensis found in goat's milk in Malta (Bruce).
1887—Meningococcus (Weichselbaum).
1894—Plague bacillus (Kitasato and Yersin).
1905—Treponema pallidum of syphilis (Schaudinn).

The importance of the discovery of these bacilli and the proof of their causal relation to the respective diseases did not consist merely in their rendering accurate diagnosis possible, and in the establishment of public health laboratories for this and allied purposes.

Pasteur led the way in endeavours to inoculate animals with attenuated bacteria, rendered less virulent by special methods of laboratory culture. His work in protecting sheep against anthrax is well known; as is also his success, without having isolated its causal agent, in inoculating persons bitten by a mad dog or wolf with emulsions from specially treated spinal cords of rabic rabbits. In working on these lines he was inspired by Jenner's success against small-pox, but as already noted (p. 175) more recent successes in producing temporary immunity have been the result of inoculation with dead cultures of the respective bacilli in typhoid fevers, in diphtheria, and possibly in scarlet fever. In diphtheria Von Behring and Roux led the way in saving life in early attacks of the disease by an antitoxin. Immunity against this disease is now obtainable by a mixed toxin and antitoxin.

Theobald Smith (1859–   ) in 1886 shewed that

immunity from hog cholera is conferred by injecting into susceptible animals the filtrate of the specific organisms.

Bordet's, Von Behring's, and Metschnikoff's work came later, and the investigation of immunity is still being assiduously pursued for various diseases. Unhappily little or no success has hitherto been attained in protecting mankind against the acute respiratory infections—influenza, pneumonia, bronchitis,—which are chief causes of premature death.

From this hasty glance at some of the outstanding discoveries in preventive medicine since 1870, we may turn to the vast increase of our power of control of tropical and sub-tropical diseases. Here again Theobald Smith blazed a new path, by shewing the need for an intermediate host—a tick—in the causation and spread of Texas Fever, and thus pointed to a new direction for the investigation of certain communicable diseases. This was in 1889.

A momentous advance in our knowledge of intermediate hosts of parasites was made by Patrick Manson (1844–1922), when he shewed that the filaria sanguinis hominis discovered by T. Lewis in 1872 only migrated into the blood circulation of human carriers at night; that mosquitoes sucked the blood and with it embryonic filariæ from the carrier; that the filaria becomes mature in the mosquito and is introduced into a new human host when he is bitten by it.

This was followed by the epoch making investigations of Ronald Ross (1857–   ) on malaria, in relation to mosquitoes; shewing that by exterminating mosquitoes in and about houses, by screening patients and others at night, and by allied measures, malaria may be made to cease out of the earth; if all would assist in carrying out the measures which demonstrably will effect this.

This led to the dramatic demonstration by Walter Reed (1851–1902) and his collaborators, anticipated in certain particulars by Henry R. Carter, that yellow fever is communicated to man by the bite of a special variety of mosquito, the stegomya. Yellow fever is now more nearly extinct in its old haunts than is typhus fever in crowded city communities.

This chapter would swell to undue proportions if one did more than enumerate ankylostomiasis, yaws, tropical sleeping sickness, among other diseases, which as the result in the main of exact knowledge of the life history of their contagia and application of this knowledge, have been reduced in frequency or can be so reduced.

So far I have only incidentally mentioned two communicable diseases which when acquired in adequate dosage continue to ravage their hosts for long years.

Tuberculosis has pestered mankind as far back as medical records exist. Laennec (1781–1826) taught that every case of phthisis develops from tubercles. Villemin, in 1865, shewed the inoculability of matter from tubercles, and formulated the statement that tuberculosis is caused by a specific virus. Koch's discovery of the tubercle bacillus in 1882 opened the way for exact knowledge of this disease and its methods of spread both in animals and man. Whether any prophylactic or curative vaccine will become available for this disease is still doubtful. Meanwhile there is no question as to the preventability of tuberculosis, by precautionary measures which are easily practicable.

The prospects of eliminating syphilis are more immediate than those for tuberculosis; because a specific means of treatment has been discovered, and because—apart from congenital syphilis and accidental syphilis—syphilis is only acquired as the direct result of impure sexual congress. The universal adoption of a standard of conduct which would eliminate promiscuity would wipe out this disease, as well as gonorrhoea, in a couple of generations.

In 1903 Metchnikoff and Roux first inoculated monkeys with syphilis; in 1905 Schaudinn discovered the Treponema pallidum in primary lesions; in 1906 Neisser, Bruck, and Wassermann introduced the serological test in diagnosis; and in 1910 Ehrlich discovered salvarsan.

Allusion should be made in conclusion to certain physical and physiological discoveries which are widening the scope of preventive medicine.

The work of Flügge, of Haldane, and of Leonard Hill, has demonstrated the importance of movement of air and of avoidance of excessive humidity in the ventilation of rooms. The older stress laid on the amount of carbonic acid in rooms we now know is only justified in so far as this gives some rough index of the likelihood of infection from person to person.

Recent work on the value of ultra-violet radiations of light in the prevention and treatment of rickets is most important; and the irradiation of milk as an additional means of ultra-violet therapy and hygiene opens out great possibilities of improved health.

Reference may also be made to the discovery of vitamins or accessory food substances, which will probably render specific starvation of essential elements in the dietary a thing of the past.

Scurvy was eliminated before the anti-scorbutic vitamin was found; just as typhus in most countries had been eliminated before its exact method of spread —by body lice—had been ascertained. But the discovery of these essential elements in food renders it possible to give exactitude to measures which previously might be compared to an old-fashioned medical prescription including many drugs, only one of which is the real therapeutic agent. The discovery of vitamins should not, however, lead to the unjustifiable conclusion that an adequate and well balanced dietary has become less important.

INDEX OF PROPER NAMES

Anson, Admiral, 192
Aristotle, 14, 25
Armstrong, G., 61, 206
Asclepiads, 11
Auenbrugger, 53
Augustine, St., 9
Avenzoar, 163
Avicenna, 69

Bacon, Francis, 24, 26, 35, 103
Bacon, Roger, 17, 24
Baillie, Matthew, 53
Baker, George, 42
Barlow, T., 210
Bascome, 62
Bateman, T., 170
Behring, Von, 215, 216
Bentham, J., 116
Berkeley, Bishop, 156
Bernard, Claude, 55
Bichat, 53
Blane, G., 110, 192
Boccaccio, 59
Boerhaave, 31, 63
Boghurst, W., 76
Bordet, 216
Boyle, Robert, 9, 37, 39, 84
Bretonneau, 54, 129
Bristowe, J. S., 127
Broussais, 53, 64
Brown, John, 63
Browne, Sir Thomas, 9, 16
Budd, William, 139, 146, 160

Cadogan, W., 206
Calmette, 175
Carlyle, T., 110
Carter, H. R., 217
Cavendish, 38
Celsas, 59
Chadwick, Edwin, 106, 116, 137, 149
Chamberlin, 181
Chapin, C. V., 67
Chereau, 77
Cook, Captain, 42, 192
Copernicus, 36
Crawford, R., 9, 29
Cullen, 51, 63
Currie, 108

Davis, J. B., 206
Davy, H., 41
Da Vinci, Leonardo, 28
Digby, Kenelm, 35
Dimsdale, 170
Duclaux, 54

Ehrlich, 218
Elliott, J. S., 89
Esculapius, 11

Farr, William, 68, 114, 150, 153
Ferriar, John, 108
Flügge, 218
Fothergill, J., 114, 173
Frascatorius, 69

Galen, 12, 14, 21, 59, 65
Galileo, 21, 36
Galvani, 36
Garrison, F. H., vii, 2, 18, 56, 69, 163
Garrod, A., 34
Gerhard, 129
Gilbert, W., 36
Glisson, 211
Gordon, A., 183
Graunt, John, 113
Guy, W. A., 192

Hahnemann, 50
Haldane, J. S., 218
Hales, Stephen, 105, 193
Halley, 9
Hancock, 73
Harvey, Wm., 1, 23, 26, 29, 181
Hawkins, R., 192
Haygarth, J., 107, 170, 172
Heberden, W., 74, 172
Herodotus, 7
Hill, Leonard, 218
Hippocrates, 4, 11, 13, 34, 57, 65
Hodge, N., 77
Hoffmann, 51
Holmes, O. W., 156, 183
Howard, John, 98, 106, 109,
Hunter, John, 53, 176
Huxham, 42

James, 94
Jenner, Edward, 176
Jenner, Sir William, 86, 129

Kingsley, C., 93
Kircher, 69
Koch, R., 214

Laennec, 52, 188, 217
Latour, C., 86
Lavoisier, 37, 38
Leeuwenhoek, 39
Lewis, T., 216
Liebig, 86
Lind, James, 106, 159, 194
Lister, J. J., 39
Lister, Lord, 179, 189, 214
Locke, John, 83
Louis, 84, 129
Lower, 37
Ludwig, 55
Luther, Martin, 9

Malpighi, 37
Malthus, 97
Mandeville H. de, 180
Manson, P., 216
Mapother, 90, 94, 157,
Martin, 100
Mayow, 37
Mead, R., 78, 83, 122, 193
Meigs, C. L., 184
Metschnikoff, 216, 218
Miethe, 22
Molière, 51
Montagu, Lady, 170
Moon, R. O., 15
Morgagni, 52
Morley, John, 51
Muller, Johannes, 55
Murchison, C., 86, 127, 132, 188

Newton, I, 9
Nightingale, F., 106

Origen, 9

Palmerston, 10
Paracelsus, 21, 31, 35, 179
Pare, Ambroise, 78, 181
Parkin, J., 60
Pasteur, ix, 175, 213
Payne, J. F., 33, 65, 67
Percival, Thomas, 50, 108, 114, 170
Perkin, 41
Pettenkofer, 142, 147
Plato, 13
Priestley, 37, 38
Pringle, J., 70, 103, 163
Purchas, 194

Raleigh, W., 192
Rawlinson, R., 89, 90
Reed, Walter, 217
Rhazes, 68, 155, 168
Richardson, B. W., 115, 142
Ridi, Francesco, 85
Romilly, 111
Ross, Ronald, 216
Rousseau, 84
Roux, 215
Rush, B., 50, 135
Russell, J. Burn, 92
Russell, Lord J., 119

Salerno, School of, 18
Sanderson, Burdon, 55
Schaudinn, 218
Schwann, T., 86, 214
Sedgwick, W. T., 143
Semmelweis, 183, 185
Shaftesbury, Lord, 106
Shattuck, Jemuel, 94
Simon, John, 2, 96, 110, 136, 143, 152
Singer, C and S., 69
Smith, Adam, 97
Smith, Hugh, 209
Smith, Southwood, 106, 116, 119, 121, 125, 137, 149
Smith, Theobald, 214, 216
Smyth, C., 159
Snow, John, 136, 142, 145
Spallanzani, 39
Stewart, A. P., 129
Stokes, W., 86
Strong, R. P., 164
Sudhoff, Karl, 56
Sutton, S., 193
Swift, Dean, 89
Sydenham, 4, 30, 52, 61, 63, 66, 75, 127, 145, 162
Sylvius, 63

Takaki, K., 197
Tansillo, L., 207
Taylor, M. W., 140
Theoderic, 180
Trotter, 197

Underwood, M., 206

Vesalius, 28
Villemin, 54, 217
Virchow, 54, 188

Waterhouse, B., 173
Watson, Thomas, 86
Watt, R., 169
Welch, W. H., vi, 21, 28, 50, 54
Wesley, John, 97
White, C., 182
Wilberforce, W., 98, 111
Willis, T, 181
Withington, 17, 52

INDEX OF SUBJECTS

(See also Contents, pages xi–xv)

Alcohol, 199
Anatomy, 28
Anti-scorbutic prophylaxis, 193
Antiseptic surgery, 180, 214
Astrology, 16, 69
Authority and service, 23

Beri-beri, 197
Breast feeding, 210
Burial, intra-mural, 95

Chemistry and medicine, 40
Cholera, 10, 74, 141
Circulation of blood, 20
Cleanliness, 15
Climate, 67
Colic, Devonshire, 42
Compulsion in scurvy, 196
Contagion, see Infection
Contagionists, 80
Cruelty to animals, 100
Cyclical influences, 71

Deductive reasoning, 25
Disinfectants, 146
Disinfection, 154, 187
Disinfestation, 164
Doctrine, 7, 50
Dysentery, 104

Economics and health, 115
Effluvia, 136, 157
Epidemic Constitution, 65, 127
Epidemiology, 32, 63
Ethics, 13

Famine, 190
Fasting for Cholera, 10
Fermentations, 85, 213
"Fever," 121
Fever hospitals, 107
Food poisoning, 200
Food sophistication, 201
Foundling hospitals, 209

Ground water, 153

Housing, 91
Humanitarian movement, 98
Hypothesis, 7, 64

Immunity, 66
Immunization, 215
Inductive reasoning, 26
Infantile hygiene, 203
Infection, 56, 63
Influenza, 71, 168
Inoculation, 166
Intermediate hosts, 216

King's Evil, 9

Lead poisoning, 43
Lemon juice, 194
Leprosy, 57
Lice, 132

Listerism, 180, 189
Localists, 80

Miasma, 126
Microscope, 39
Midwifery forceps, 181
Milk and fever, 139
Mortality, bills of, 113

Observation in medicine, 31

Pandemics, 71
Parasites, 216
Pathology, 52
Plague, 58, 72, 75
Poor-law reform, 98, 116
Potato, 191
Poverty, 113
Predisposition, 145
Prison reform, 106
Puerperal sepsis, 182
Pythogenic fever, 138

Rats and plague, 82
Registration of deaths, 113, 204
Respiration, 37
Rickets, 203, 206, 211

Sacerdotalism, 7
Sanitation, 88
Scabies, 162
Science and medicine, 34
Scurvy, 191
Season and disease, 65
Segregation, 122
Sepsis, 179
Sewerage, 90
Shell-fish, 134
Small pox, 68, 71, 166
Smoke nuisance, 93
Social betterment, 97
Soil and disease, 148
Spontaneous generation, 85
Supernaturalism, 11
Syphilis, 203, 218

Theory, 7
Trench fever, 133
Tuberculosis, 53, 217
Typhoid fever, 86, 102, 129
Typhus fever, 71, 100, 109, 129, 131

Vaccination, 171, 175
Ventilation, 105, 218

Water supplies, 90, 143
Wesleyan revival, 111
Wet nurses, 207
Window tax, 95
Witchcraft, 16

Yellow fever, 134, 217

Zymotic diseases, 68

Sans Tache

WAVERLY PRESS INCORPORATED · BALTIMORE ·

SANS TACHE

Sans Tache

IN THE "elder days of art" each artist or craftsman enjoyed the privilege of independent creation. He carried through a process of manufacture from beginning to end. The scribe of the days before the printing press was such a craftsman. So was the printer in the days before the machine process. He stood or fell, as a craftsman, by the merit or demerit of his finished product.

Modern machine production has added much to the worker's productivity and to his material welfare; but it has deprived him of the old creative distinctiveness. His work is merged in the work of the team, and lost sight of as something representing him and his personality.

Many hands and minds contribute to the manufacture of a book, in this day of specialization. There are seven distinct major processes in the making of a book: The type must first be set; by the monotype method, there are two processes, the "keyboarding" of the MS and the casting of the type from the perforated paper rolls thus produced. Formulas and other intricate work must be hand-set; then the whole brought together ("composed") in its true order, made into pages and forms. The results must be checked by proof reading at each stage. Then comes the "make-ready" and press-run and finally the binding into volumes.

All of these processes, except that of binding into cloth or leather covers, are carried on under our roof.

The motto of the Waverly Press is *Sans Tache.* Our ideal is to manufacture books "*without blemish*"—worthy books, worthily printed, with worthy typography—books to which we shall be proud to attach our imprint, made by craftsmen who are willing to accept open responsibility for their work, and who are entitled to credit for creditable performance.

The printing craftsman of today is quite as much a craftsman as his predecessor. There is quite as much discrimination between poor work and good. We are of the opinion that the individuality of the worker should not be wholly lost. The members of our staff who have contributed their skill of hand and brain to this volume are:

Composing: Ernest Salgado, William E. Fite, James Armiger, John Flanagan, Austin Uhland, William Sanders, Arthur Baker, James Jackson, Edgar Simmons, Anthony Wagner, John Crabill, Nathan Miller, Andrew Rassa, Herbert C. Leitch, Edward Rice, Richard King, George Moss, Theodore Nilson, Henry Shea.

Caster: Kenneth Brown, Charles Aher, Ernest Wann, Mahlon Robinson, George Smith, Henry Lee, Martin Griffen, Charles Fick, George Bullinger, Frank Malanosky.

Keyboard: Vera Taylor, Helen Twardowicz, Anna Rustic, Hannah Scott, Mildred Lambert.

Press: Fred Lucker, Henry Augsburg.

Folder: Laurence Krug, Shipley Dellinger.

Proof Room: Sarah Katzin, Mary Reed, Alice Reuter, Lucille Bull, Ethel Strasinger, Ruth Treischman, Dorothy Strasinger, Ida Zimmerman, George Southworth, Angeline Eifert, Audrey Tanner, Lillian Gilland.